INFECTED

Also written and edited by Muhammad H. Zaman

We Wait for a Miracle: Health Care and the Forcibly Displaced
Bitter Pills: The Global War on Counterfeit Drugs
Biography of Resistance: The Epic Battle Between People and Pathogens
Migration and Health
Statistical Mechanics of Cellular Systems and Processes
Rah-e-Naward-e-Shoq (Urdu)
Aaina Haaye Khud Shanasi (Urdu)

INFECTED

*How Power, Politics, and Privilege Use
Science Against the World's Most Vulnerable*

* * * *

MUHAMMAD H. ZAMAN

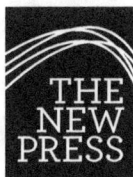

THE
NEW
PRESS

NEW YORK
LONDON

© 2025 by Muhammad H. Zaman
All rights reserved.
No part of this book may be reproduced, in any form, without written permission from the publisher.

Requests for permission to reproduce selections from this book should be made through our website: https://thenewpress.org/contact-us/.

Published in the United States by The New Press, New York, 2025
Distributed by Two Rivers Distribution

ISBN 978-1-62097-752-1 (hc)
ISBN 978-1-62097-903-7 (ebook)
CIP data is available

The New Press publishes books that promote and enrich public discussion and understanding of the issues vital to our democracy and to a more equitable world. These books are made possible by the enthusiasm of our readers; the support of a committed group of donors, large and small; the collaboration of our many partners in the independent media and the not-for-profit sector; booksellers, who often hand-sell New Press books; librarians; and above all by our authors.

www.thenewpress.org

Printed in the United States of America

10 9 8 7 6 5 4 3 2 1

For Afreen, Rahem and Samah

Contents

Prologue

By the time she reached the border, Maria knew that the baby was due any day.[1] Since leaving her home in Honduras over three months ago, she, her husband, and her toddler son had walked for days, hitched rides on the back of trucks, and walked again. The threats from the local gang, MS-13, had become specific and targeted at her husband. Maria knew she had to act quickly. She had lost close family members in the preceding few months to the gang violence that had engulfed her country.

With meager possessions that could be packed in small bags, the family of three had set out in late 2019, believing that they had a credible case for asylum in the United States. The journey was difficult and took longer than expected, not only because they had little money and were under constant threat of violence but also because Maria was pregnant and not doing too well.

Maria and her family reached the Texas border in late March of 2020. As soon as they arrived, they were detained and then taken to a U.S. Border Patrol facility. By this time, Maria was already having stomach pains and was in a bad state. Soon her water broke, and she was taken to a local hospital in Rio Grande Valley. Despite exhaustion and malnutrition, Maria gave birth to a healthy baby girl.

Two days later, Maria, along with her newborn, was discharged, handed back to the border patrol officials, and reunited with the rest of the family. Maria was hopeful that their asylum case would move forward and they would soon be able to live in the United States, far away from the constant threat of violence in her hometown. But they were never brought in front of an asylum judge. Instead, just days after the birth of their daughter, while Maria was still recovering, they were taken to an international bridge and forced to walk to Mexico. It wasn't that their asylum case was denied but that they were not even entitled to apply for asylum. Shocked at this treatment, Maria and her family tried to protest and seek answers. They were told there was nothing they could do. The rules had changed recently, and asylum was no longer an option, no matter how strong their case was.

Maria and her family were deemed a threat to U.S. public health. Later on, Maria would learn that she was denied her right to asylum by a U.S. law few had heard of. It was called Title 42.[2]

Months later, when Maria spoke to reporters from a tiny apartment in Mexico, a country she was unfamiliar with, she felt a deep sense of loss. She had left Honduras before the first case of the pandemic had been reported. She and her whole family had never had COVID-19. Even at the hospital where she gave birth, none of the doctors or nurses suspected that she had been exposed to the virus. She simply could not understand why she was considered a threat to anyone's health.

Maria also felt a sense of betrayal and injustice. Her daughter was born in the United States, and she had paperwork from the hospital to prove it. Technically, her daughter was a U.S. citizen, but the paperwork and Maria's protest did not matter to the border agents who told her to march south to Mexico. In a similar case with another Honduran family, recognizing that the baby was born in the United States and hence a U.S. citizen, the Customs and Border Protection (CBP) authorities made an offer to the mother. The mother had to leave the United States no matter what. But if she chose, she could give up her two-day-old baby to child services in the United States.[3] The mother, shocked at the offer, refused and deported herself and the family to Mexico.

Similar stories emerged in other parts of the country. One woman who had a C-section was sent to Mexico within a week of her surgery.[4] She could barely walk, and most of her wounds had not yet healed. In other cases, moms and babies were sent back to cities like Tijuana that continue to face the challenges of homicide, kidnapping, and brutal gang violence—places very similar to what these families had escaped from in the first place. Only this time it was in a new country.

* * * *

INFECTION'S RELATIONSHIP WITH political decision-making is long and tragic, and the aim of this book is to analyze how infection, or infectious disease research, has been co-opted by states and state-affiliated agencies in ways that harm society's most vulnerable members. This has nothing to do with casting doubt on the efficacy of vaccines, or imagining that vaccines cause autism, or that one should not trust science. The central argument is, in fact, quite the opposite. It is about how good science, discovery, and knowledge are used for political purposes.

The episodes of exploitation of infectious disease research fall into three main categories, although it is important to recognize that the categories overlap. The first category is the use of infection to enact exclusionary policies, such as the Chinese Exclusion Act of 1882 and Title 42 during the COVID-19 pandemic. Time and again, infection has been used to stigmatize individuals and communities that those in power distrust, even when scientific evidence suggested no connection between these groups and the disease. Skin color, religion, and national origin have all been linked to infectious disease. In part, this is because foreigners and ethnic minorities are often socioeconomically disadvantaged, and it has been easy to make the connection between poverty and infectious disease. Add to that the inherent racism and xenophobia that have allowed many to accept that certain groups are by nature unhygienic and hence a source of disease for the majority communities.

This stigmatization of poorer minority communities has resulted in their forced exclusion from the labor market and their expulsion from towns, cities, and even countries. Wrapped within the cloak of proactive public health and infection control, this approach of stigmatization based on national origin and ethnicity has been a powerful tool, as it claims that the government action is for public welfare and safety. It has found support not just in the court of public opinion but also in actual courts of justice that have summarily rejected challenges and lawsuits questioning the legality of such policies. The Chinese and the Irish in the late nineteenth and early twentieth centuries, and others deemed outsiders, have all borne the brunt of these campaigns. Even when the scientific community or epidemiologists rejected the premise on which these campaigns are based or questioned their limited and selective use of data, the campaigns have continued at full pace.

The second way nations, including but not limited to the United States, have deployed infection is by harming vulnerable groups in the name of the greater good of society or scientific discovery. The German East African sleeping sickness campaign, the Tuskegee syphilis study, and the Guatemala gonorrhea experiments are relevant examples here. In these situations, ideas rooted in racism have been put into practice and the vulnerabilities of the community have been exploited contrary to the fundamental ethical principles of medicine and public health. Communities deemed racially or morally inferior have been deliberately held back from adequate, accessible care. Historically marginalized communities have been exposed to pathogens or given a disease without their consent or without appropriate treatment, in federally sponsored programs, all in the name of scientific progress.

The third dimension is the use of infection and infectious disease research for national security purposes—that is, the actual weaponization of infection. The development of biological weapons and the fake public health campaigns in Pakistan (discussed in chapter 1) illustrate this dimension. Those in charge of supporting the development of biological weapons knew full well that these instruments of war would affect ordinary, unsuspecting citizens in foreign lands. In fact, this was the explicit goal. Soldiers are probably more likely to be prepared and capable of taking evasive action or protecting themselves than are civilians, who include the elderly, children, and the disabled. Infectious agents, developed meticulously through careful research and released through the air or transported through waterways, can stay in the environment for a long period and be carried to towns and cities over a vast geography. Unlike the traditional weapons of war that might target communication and transport infrastructure or military installations, biological weapons are explicitly meant to cause maximum damage by killing and maiming people and by overwhelming hospitals. Above all, they are meant to cause widespread panic and terror. Biological weapons are the deliberate product of a process in which scientific discoveries have been co-opted for harm, not welfare. In this case, weapons are made from the scientific knowledge about pathogens and toxins and how they overwhelm the natural defenses of the body, destroy the nervous system, or lead to complete paralysis. This knowledge, combined with the ability to package anthrax or ricin, rests on a deeper understanding of how to use the appropriate materials to store and release these toxins and how to make the toxins potent for maximum efficiency.

This book focuses on the events in the last 150 years, primarily because of a major scientific and technological shift that occurred in the second half of the nineteenth century.[5] The arrival of the germ theory of disease, developed during this period, changed the world of infectious diseases forever. In the last hundred years, the discovery of antibiotics, the development of vaccines, the design of rapid diagnostics, and the advancement of population-level infection control methods have saved millions, if not hundreds of millions, of lives. It is also important to note that many forms of technology were not developed for the purposes of weaponization or exploitation, but their availability made weaponization possible. We cannot ignore the fact that deliberate instances of exploiting the legitimate scientific discoveries surrounding infectious disease have increased. One would have expected that some of the previous ideas and policies that weaponized infection and exploited marginalized communities would have ended by now. But that has not happened. In fact, existing policies have continued despite scientific evidence that disproves perceived links between race and disease.[6] And in other instances, such as Title 42 enactment, new policies were created in light of disease outbreaks. In repeated instances, power, privilege, and prejudice have become the dominant drivers in co-opting good research for political purposes. This book is an attempt to understand how legitimate research and novel discoveries in infectious diseases, while saving millions of lives, have also fueled harmful political agendas.

Between the late nineteenth century and up to the writing of this text, the list of instances in which research on infectious diseases was used by various governments and strong political entities for specific unethical purposes is long. I view the impact of these episodes to be both vertical and horizontal: vertical in the sense that one event, practice, or idea fed the next and continued over time; horizontal because one community, institution, or country copied it and modified it to suit unique local circumstances. These aspects cannot be viewed as an isolated series of incidents and events but instead need to be studied and analyzed as part of a single continuum.

This book does not seek to discuss each and every episode of the weaponization or exploitation of infection in the last 150 years. The selection is meant to be illustrative rather than comprehensive. Much has been written on the individual episodes I describe, including outstanding books, rich in detail and sophisticated in analysis, by historians, public health experts, journalists, and other researchers. I have benefited tremendously from this scholarship. Unlike these other studies, this book aims to connect several episodes of weaponization and exploitation with the scientific and technological developments of the time and to analyze how the latest technologies were utilized for political goals. This book also focuses on the ways these episodes are interconnected. At the same time, this book discusses how particular political goals fueled investments in developing new technologies in diagnosing and managing infection.

From a scientific and clinical standpoint, the arguments in the book focus specifically on infection and infectious disease research. Unethical practices rooted in racism and xenophobia around noncommunicable diseases, such as the treatment of those with cancer or cognitive disabilities, the intentional denial of care to the vulnerable during pregnancy, and the underfunding of hospitals in historically marginalized communities, while incredibly important to study, are outside the scope of this book.[7] Similarly, the repeated and frequent targeting of health care workers, ambulances, and health facilities with weapons developed in countries with flourishing defense industries is also not the focus of this book.

This book makes a case for viewing these overlapping episodes and distinct strategies as part of a weaponization-exploitation continuum. Whether it is the actual development of a weapon, or the use of infection to stigmatize or expel a particular ethnic group, or the unethical testing of toxins on a particular community, or the use of infection control as a means of gathering intelligence, these strategies all represent the same goal: using science and research meant for the greater good of humanity to harm the disenfranchised, weak, and vulnerable.

1

The Campaigns

THE PICTURE THAT WENT VIRAL WAS TAKEN AT
4:05 p.m. on May 1, 2011. The president of the United States,
wearing a black jacket, is looking intently at a screen that is not
visible in the picture. The vice president is sitting next to the president. At the head of the table, looking down and working on his
computer, is a U.S. Air Force general. On the other side of the
table is the secretary of state, her hand covering part of her face.
The group, which also includes the secretary of defense and other
officials, is in a small conference room somewhere in the White
House watching the live feed of one of the biggest moments of
President Obama's presidency: Navy SEALs are entering the compound of Osama bin Laden in Abbottabad, Pakistan.

President Obama's announcement the next day made headlines
around the world, including in my home country, Pakistan.[1] Many
Pakistanis, including those in my immediate family, were surprised,
shocked, and uncertain as to what to make of the whole episode.
The government of Pakistan was both furious and embarrassed.[2]
Furious because it believed that its territorial sovereignty was
breached and that a foreign power carried out a military operation
on its soil without permission. Embarrassed because Osama bin
Laden, the most wanted man in the world at the time, was found
in a residential compound just a few miles from the highly secure

Pakistan Military Academy. The episode has shaped U.S.- Pakistan relations in the years since. It also started a global conversation about the influence of politics and power on efforts for infectious disease eradication.[3]

Twenty days after bin Laden was killed, a local doctor, Shakeel Afridi, was arrested by Pakistan's military intelligence.[4] Authorities accused Dr. Afridi of helping the CIA by running a fake hepatitis B vaccination campaign in Abbottabad. The details of when and how Afridi first came in contact with the CIA are murky, but sometime in early 2011, the CIA and its local operatives recruited him for a clandestine mission. By that time, the CIA had a strong suspicion that bin Laden was living in or around the city of Abbottabad in northwest Pakistan. There were still several gaps in intelligence, and many within the CIA were skeptical. Stronger evidence was needed to convince the naysayers. One way to get that evidence and close the gap in intelligence was to match the DNA of those living in the compound, presumably bin Laden's children, with that of bin Laden's sister, who had died in 2010 in Boston.[5] The CIA put this long-shot operation in motion and hired Afridi to run a fake vaccination campaign with the hope of gathering the bin Laden family's DNA.

Since the residents of the compound where bin Laden was supposedly living rarely came out or interacted with their neighbors or the community at large, getting the children's DNA was not a straightforward operation. To acquire what they needed, CIA agents concocted an elaborate plan. It created a large campaign promising free hepatitis B vaccines in Abbottabad. Hepatitis B—a vaccine-preventable viral disease—is common in Pakistan, as well as in a number of low- and middle-income countries.[6] It is estimated that there are several million hepatitis B patients in Pakistan.[7] Given the high burden of infectious diseases, vaccine campaigns are fairly common in Pakistan and are often funded by international donors, as funding for health care has never been a government priority.[8] The government is glad to outsource such campaigns to outsiders who are willing to foot the bill and create jobs for local health care professionals. Yet despite international involvement, public health campaigns in Pakistan still require several levels of government approval and significant paperwork. These approvals take a lot of time, sometimes years, before the actual programs can be rolled out.

Since no vaccination campaign for the region had been approved by the national or local governments in 2010 or 2011, Afridi bribed the low-ranking government officials in Abbottabad to bypass the necessary paperwork needed for a vaccine drive. Corruption is rampant in the country and bribes are not unheard of, so no one bothered to ask why Afridi, who was a surgeon and who was not a hepatitis specialist or an expert in running vaccination campaigns, was in charge of this new initiative. In addition, no questions were asked about the fact that Afridi was also not from Abbottabad and had no personal or professional reason to be in the city.

With funds from the CIA, posters promoting the virtues and necessity of vaccines were quickly printed and put up around Abbottabad.[9] The vaccination campaign started in March 2011. After the necessary fanfare and promotion, the first vaccination sites were carefully chosen to be in the poor neighborhoods of the city to make the campaign look believable. Free vaccination campaigns in urban slums are not unusual in Pakistan. Like many other parts of the world, the burden of infection is disproportionately high among the poorer neighborhoods in Pakistan, especially in crowded informal settlements and slums that lack basic health infrastructure and sanitation systems. Local doctors have little incentive to work in these places, and the government often relies on foreign NGOs to provide essential public health services in these communities, including vaccinations.

The goal of this campaign, however, was neither to vaccinate children nor to prevent the awful disease.[10] After operating in the impoverished part of the city for just a few weeks, the campaign quickly and abruptly moved to Bilal Town in April 2011. Bilal Town is in a more affluent part of the city, away from the poor neighborhoods and barely a kilometer from the main entrance of the heavily guarded Pakistan Military Academy—the main training facility for young recruits who join the ranks of the military as officers. Bilal Town is also where the CIA believed bin Laden had been living for some time. Since no one was monitoring the campaign or was aware of its plans, no questions were asked about why the focus was shifted suddenly, before the completion of the vaccine drive in the slums. The poor children, who were promised three doses of the vaccine, never got more than one. Some did not even get the first dose.

With the campaign closer to its real goal, it was time to start the next phase of the mission. The team had to, somehow, get a blood sample from the children living in the compound. Vaccination— as anyone who has gotten a shot in the arm can attest to—does not typically lead to the drawing of blood. A new plan was, therefore, hatched to get a few drops of blood, without causing any suspicion among the children or their caregivers. A local nurse, Mukhtar Bibi, was hired to vaccinate and simultaneously draw blood from the children in the compound. Bibi maintains, to this day, that she was never told the real purpose of the campaign and that she was hired only to be the public health worker who would vaccinate against hepatitis B.[11] Whether she asked why she was drawing blood during routine vaccination—and if she did ask, what answers she was provided—is still unknown. As she prepared to give the first dose of the vaccine (and draw blood), she was provided a handbag. The handbag not only had the necessary medical tools but was fitted with an electronic device. Bibi, in later interviews, insisted that she had no idea about the device.

The details of what happened next are murky and still shrouded in secrecy. No one from the region I spoke to, including physicians, nurses, and community workers, wanted to talk about the episode.

What is known, however, is that the elaborate but phony vaccination campaign was a failure. It provided no valuable intelligence.

* * * *

SOON AFTER THE Abbottabad operation that killed bin Laden in May 2011, Pakistani intelligence agencies were able to track down Dr. Afridi and learn more about the supposed hepatitis vaccination campaign. He was quickly put behind bars. In a society where anti-American sentiment had been brewing for quite some time, the public's anger at the raid to get bin Laden was palpable.[12] Afridi was viewed as a traitor by many in Pakistan for helping the CIA. But doubts lingered in large sections of the society. A number of questions were being asked all across the country, including in my own family: Was bin Laden actually hiding in Abbottabad?[13] If so, for how long? Did a Pakistani doctor actually help the CIA? Was it money or something else that forced him to become a "traitor"? Who else knew about it? Was the government complicit or complacent? Was the vaccination campaign actually a fraud? Should we be skeptical about other public health campaigns funded by international donors?[14] What else—under the guise of public health and welfare—is going on that we do not know about?

The doubts about whether the CIA campaign was real or fictional were put to rest, not by a newspaper story or a well-connected investigative journalist but by the U.S. secretary of defense. Leon Panetta, in a *60 Minutes* interview aired on January 29, 2012, spoke openly about the CIA operation.[15] Mr. Panetta showed no remorse or regrets for creating a fake vaccination campaign. On the contrary, he was surprised and angry that there would be such a reaction in Pakistan against one of its citizens who was so useful to the CIA. He showed no concern or interest for public health or what the vaccination campaign might have meant for the people of Pakistan. "For them to take this kind of action against somebody who was helping to go after terrorism, I just think is a real mistake on their part," he said emphatically.[16]

The impact of the fake vaccination campaign on the local community in Pakistan, however, was significant and long lasting. Pakistan's support for the United States in the war on terror was already widely unpopular, and strong anti-U.S. sentiment was present throughout the country.[17] In the northwest of the country, drone attacks and local instability had wreaked havoc on millions of lives.[18] Thousands of people had lost loved ones. Among those who died were men, women, and children who had nothing to do with the Taliban, al-Qaeda, or the Pakistani government. They were ordinary people who just happened to live in a particular part of the country. Families were affected by life-changing and permanently disabling injuries and the loss of livelihood. The psychological trauma of drone attacks affected entire communities.[19] The word *drone* became synonymous with surveillance, anxiety, and possible destruction. The revelations that the CIA had manufactured a phony public health campaign for a U.S. national security mission further fueled anger against the United States and Western nations. The ruse further underscored the lingering idea among people in Pakistan that only some lives matter, and that people in poorer parts of the world are expendable on the altar of rich nations' politics. These sentiments of anger and frustration strengthened the local anti-U.S. and anti-Western political and militant groups that already had a strong base in the region. The local Taliban groups, unsurprisingly, were among the biggest beneficiaries of the fake vaccination campaign.[20] The changing situation, and strong anti-American sentiment combined with mistrust of public health efforts, strengthened their bargaining power. They used it as an excuse to stop all other vaccination efforts by the government, calling them a continuation of the CIA's activities in the country and an effort by another country to undermine the independence and sovereignty of the people.

While the local political groups benefited from the situation, ordinary Pakistanis, who were already suffering from the combined effects of poverty, government apathy, high infection rates, and low public spending on health, paid a heavy price for the U.S.-sponsored fake hepatitis vaccination campaign. The biggest casualty of this episode was the national effort to eradicate polio.[21] The polio eradication campaign was now widely viewed with suspicion by the local population and was considered an extension of the CIA campaign. Soon, it became the target of public anger, and local tribal and religious leadership exploited the growing distrust for their own political gains.

* * * *

BY THE EARLY 2000s, Pakistan was among the last few countries with polio, and it was on track to eliminate the disease in the coming years.[22] The events of early 2011 changed the downward trend of polio infections so drastically that in 2014 more than three-quarters of the world's polio cases were found in Pakistan.[23] Polio workers who were tasked with administering oral vaccines, and many of whom were women from low-income families and operated with minimal security, were attacked repeatedly. Between 2012 and 2014, sixty polio workers were killed across the country.[24] Scores more were injured and disabled permanently from violent attacks. Local Taliban leaders threatened not just the polio vaccination teams but also the parents of children who were scheduled to receive the vaccine. They made it clear that anyone allowing their children to be vaccinated was a part of the problem and hence a fair target for punishment. The salaries for the polio eradication workers were paltry to begin with and were often delayed for extended periods of time because of lack of funds, poor management, corruption, and layers of stifling government bureaucracy.[25] With frequent attacks on the vaccination teams, it became even more challenging for the government to recruit workers who were willing to take such risks. The campaign to eradicate polio started to collapse from within.

Soon, the impact on the polio eradication was no longer limited to the northwest region of the country, where the Taliban had a strong foothold and where Abbottabad is located. It was seen in towns and cities across the country. Even in big cities like Karachi, on the southernmost tip of the country and over 1,500 kilometers from Abbottabad, the distrust of the polio campaign and other vaccinations was palpable. The security situation resulted in several local polio campaigns getting derailed or suspended.[26] These suspended vaccination campaigns then resulted in a resurgence of the disease, and the sharp uptick continued for years to come. Local religious leaders, even those who had strong ideological differences with the Taliban, argued that the polio resurgence in the country was due to the CIA.[27]

The local militant groups also recognized that they now had a bargaining chip and asked for all kinds of steep concessions from the government in exchange for restarting the polio campaign or allowing other vaccination teams to operate in the regions they controlled. The public's distrust affected other international institutions and organizations that focused on infection control, disease awareness, and prevention and management, including some that had been working in the country for decades. On June 11, 2015, Save the Children, an international organization that had been working in the country since 1979 and had nearly 1,200 employees, was told that it could no longer operate in the country.[28] The offices were shut down and padlocked, and the foreign employees were given two weeks to leave the country.

* * * *

PAKISTAN'S POLIO ERADICATION effort, while being the most prominent, was not the only public health effort that was damaged in the country. Efforts to combat other preventable infectious diseases were hit hard as well. The CIA campaign came not only at a time of heightened national anxiety and anti-U.S. sentiment but also in a country where distrust of Western medicine is rife and access to quality health care is out of reach for many.[29] Large sections of Pakistani society are suspicious of Western medicine, and vaccines in particular have long been associated with a foreign conspiracy to sterilize children, cause infertility in women, or cause inexplicable illnesses.[30] The government's efforts to tackle misinformation have often been weak and ineffective. In the aftermath of the CIA campaign, social media further amplified the antivaccination voices. In the minds of those who were already suspicious of Western medicine, and of those who, perhaps, were confused about whether vaccines are good or bad, there was hard evidence to support an antivaccine agenda. Public health gains made in Pakistan over decades were quickly wiped out. New efforts, such as those to combat drug-resistant typhoid infections—another potentially deadly disease that disproportionately affects those in low-income areas—were met with stiff resistance from the local communities.[31] This trend continued for years, and during the COVID-19 pandemic, Pakistan faced, once again, strong local resistance to vaccination.[32]

By the time the country rolled out the COVID-19 vaccination campaign, few were specifically talking about the Afridi–bin Laden episode, but they did not need to. The antivaccine sentiment that was fertilized by the CIA campaign had developed deep roots of its own. In a society where public health is underfunded, frustration over the West's interference in internal matters of the country is high, and public engagement on scientific literacy has never been a priority for the government or the many NGOs that work in the country, skepticism against the COVID-19 vaccine found a rich and fertile environment. The fake hepatitis campaign—rolled out a decade before the pandemic—was still bearing fruit.[33] With widespread misinformation now available through social media, theories that denied the pandemic outright or made claims of imminent death from foreign-manufactured vaccines were widely circulating and had a captivated audience ready to believe these theories. These theories were no longer on the fringes of society and had become so mainstream that the minister of health, Dr. Faisal Sultan, who himself is an infectious disease physician, was repeatedly asked about their validity in television programs by well-known journalists.[34] While misinformation continued to be a challenge for many countries during COVID-19, including the United States, the problems in Pakistan were compounded by its recent history, dating back to the Abbottabad episode.

* * * *

WHEN THE NEWS first broke about the CIA's fake vaccination campaign in Pakistan, public health practitioners across the world were outraged.[35] They saw the trust that had been built over decades of painstaking work evaporate instantaneously. They saw their own life's mission and accomplishments destroyed overnight. Many infectious disease and public health experts also knew the devastating impact such unethical practices would have on the most vulnerable, including children, in countries that already had high rates of infection and weak public health systems. The issue was not limited to Pakistan, polio, or hepatitis; undermining the public's trust in health campaigns was going to make *everyone* more susceptible to disease, including communities in high-income countries. In January 2013, academic deans at a number of prominent public health schools in the United States wrote to President Obama voicing their disgust at the CIA's actions. Reflecting on what they had seen in Pakistan, they wrote that "international public health work builds peace and is one of the most constructive means by which our past, present, and future public health students can pursue a life of fulfillment and service. Please do not allow that outlet of common good to be closed to them because of political and/or security interests that ignore the type of unintended negative public health impacts we are witnessing in Pakistan."[36]

A year later, in May 2014, the White House announced an end to the CIA's operational use of any vaccination program.[37] It said that the agency would no longer seek to obtain or exploit DNA or other genetic material acquired through such programs. Ending the operational use of vaccination and the acquisition of DNA for intelligence gathering by the CIA was welcomed by public health professionals across the world. But weaponizing infection, infectious disease research, and information related to infection did not start with the campaign in Abbottabad. And it was unlikely to end with the announcement from the White House.

* * * *

THE FAKE VACCINATION campaign went against the very fundamentals of what science and research are supposed to be. It is an example of how an effective tool in infection control (vaccination) is misused for extracting information (the bin Laden family's DNA) in the service of a goal unrelated to the tool's mission (preventing hepatitis). The fake vaccination campaign also undermined the very foundations of public health practice. Vaccination is not meant to draw blood for testing or for DNA analysis. The campaign also blatantly disregarded the notions of informed consent. I eventually came to realize that all of these grand notions and values surrounding public health can become insignificant in the real-world politics. To date, we still do not know if anyone within the U.S. government who was aware of the program asked about the ethics of this campaign, protested against carrying it out, or resigned because they found it unacceptable.

The CIA campaign in Pakistan also provides a striking example of power dynamics and the application of different rules for different people and places. It is not difficult for me to imagine that a campaign like this would be unthinkable within the United States, Western Europe, or other affluent countries. But the rules were different for my country. The campaign exploited not only research and disease-eradication campaigns but also the existing weaknesses of the national system in Pakistan. The campaign recruited local doctors, who benefited from a perennial corrupt system to bribe local officials. Those who were involved in bribing local officials, were never brought to justice in Pakistan or the United States. Equally important to note is that there was little remorse from the CIA leadership when confronted in the *60 Minutes* episode, yet when there was pressure from in-country public health groups, the policy was changed. Pressure from my colleagues who are public health leaders in Pakistan or from other low-income countries would have mattered very little.

The Pakistan campaign is an example of one state using infection control and treatment programs, built on decades of research, for national security purposes, that have nothing to do with infection control or health care in another, much weaker state. This episode also exemplifies coordination between various departments of a powerful government and the partnership of that government with individuals and NGOs, all working toward a political mission in the name of national security. But the story neither starts in Pakistan nor ends there.

In June 2024, Reuters uncovered a program organized and orchestrated by the U.S. military to undermine confidence in COVID-19 vaccines and other life-saving aid in the Philippines, a country devastated by the pandemic.[38] The reason: to counter China's growing influence in the Philippines. The U.S. effort involved the impersonation of Filipinos and used social media to start an anti-vaccination campaign to sow distrust in vaccines coming from China. The Chinese-produced Sinovac vaccine (though shown to be less effective than mRNA vaccines) was approved by the World Health Organization and was the only vaccine available in the Philippines up to that point. The U.S. military was worried that China was making inroads into the country by providing an essential and lifesaving commodity. The campaign went beyond vaccines and targeted face masks and test kits coming from China. Reuters uncovered several hundred accounts on X (formerly Twitter) that created content to sow doubt about the vaccine among Filipinos. A senior official with the Department of Defense acknowledged the campaign's effort to undermine China's vaccine in the developing world. In the Philippines, a country with no capacity to produce protective equipment or vaccines, the impact was substantial. By June 2021, the vaccination rate in the Philippines was the lowest in the entire region, and the government was desperate to get more people inoculated. Only 2.1 million Filipinos had been vaccinated, against the government's target of 70 million. Yet, anxiety and worry, created in part by the anti-vaccination social media propaganda campaign created by the U.S. military, had created enough doubt in the minds of the people that they would rather risk dying from the disease than get a vaccine they no longer trusted.

Filipinos were not the only population targeted for COVID-19 vaccine scares. The United States, again using social media platforms, sowed fear among Muslims by spreading the rumor that the Sinovac vaccine contained pig gelatin and was therefore forbidden for its practitioners. Reuters found that as many as 150 of these social media accounts were run from Tampa, Florida, by U.S. Central Command or its contractors.

Troubled by the hesitation among their residents to get the vaccine, governments in Muslim countries and Islamic scholars argued that even if the vaccine contained pork products, they were allowed (or halal) since exceptions can be made in cases of saving a life.[39] But this was an uphill battle in communities where there was fear about the disease, limited knowledge about viruses and epidemics, and lack of trust in the local authorities. This was particularly true in Indonesia, the largest Muslim country, with nearly 230 million residents, where the government had to repeatedly intervene. Despite the assurance from Sinovac that the vaccine was free of porcine products, doubts among Muslims lingered. The president of Indonesia said that "there shouldn't be any concern about whether this vaccine is halal or not halal. We are in an emergency situation because of the Covid pandemic."[40] In other parts of Indonesia, in light of the hesitation about vaccines, new laws were passed that allowed people who refused vaccination to be punished. In my own country of Pakistan, I repeatedly heard the concern about the Chinese-manufactured

vaccines from a number of people who were unwilling to get inoculated. Many such fears continue to this day.

When asked about the campaign by Reuters, a senior U.S. military officer involved responded, "We weren't looking at this from a
public health perspective. We were looking at how we could drag
China through the mud."[41]

* * * *

THE TALE OF the weaponization of infection is more than a
particular fraudulent public health campaign in just one country
in Asia. It is a much bigger story of power, prejudice, and the politics of privilege. This book aims to tell that story.

2

The Exceptionalism
of Infection

INFECTION, THE INVASION AND GROWTH OF GERMS
in the body, is simultaneously a terrifying word and, perhaps
because of that, fodder for great stories. The success of movies like
Outbreak, *Quarantine*, and *Contagion* remind us that there is a
strong appetite for mysteries and thrillers about infections, epidemics, and pandemics.[1] *Outbreak* (1995) centers around a fictional
deadly Ebola-like virus called *Motaba*, which spread through
parts of California and subsequently all across the United States.
Quarantine (2008) follows a TV reporter and her cameraman
trapped in a quarantined building controlled by the Centers for
Disease Control. *Contagion* (2011) is a chilling disaster movie
that explores how society would respond to a real-life pandemic.
Movies on infection often use catchy one-word titles, dark imag-
ery, and dramatic music to build suspense and excitement underlying the great battle of human survival. Physicians are portrayed
as saviors of humanity, donning hazmat suits and risking their
lives in a rapidly collapsing world. By design, these movies focus
on a uniquely frightening aspect of infection: how an invisible and
seemingly unstoppable contagion can change, and in some cases
destroy, the whole world.

Hollywood movies are not the only art form inspired by infection. Literary works from all parts of the world have tapped this
resource repeatedly, with remarkable and perennial success.[2] Some

of the greatest writers of the last century have found inspiration in stories shaped by infection. Nobel Prize–winning Colombian author Gabriel García Márquez, one of the finest writers of the twentieth century, wrote about isolation, longing, and love in the time of cholera and captivated a global audience. *Nights of Plague*, the most recent bestseller by Turkish author and recipient of the Nobel Prize in literature in 2006, Orhan Pamuk, focuses on an epidemic outbreak in a fictional island in the waning years of the Ottoman Empire. Despite being published in 1947, *The Plague* by French philosopher and author Albert Camus has maintained its literary appeal. Italian short story writer and novelist Dino Buzzati wrote eloquently in "L'epidemia" ("The Epidemic") about infection that went beyond the literal disease, affecting only political dissidents.[3] Infection serves as a lens for viewing a society's values and our own understanding of the meaning of life. The fascination is, by no means, a phenomenon of the twentieth century. Seven hundred years earlier, Syrian poet Ibn al-Wardi's (d. 1349) poetry about plague was considered the most eloquent description of black death in the region for centuries.[4]

* * * *

SHAPED IN PART by literature and films, our imaginations often see infection in terms of conflict between good and evil, between mortality and the quest for survival in an unpredictable and hostile world.[5]

The image of infection that invokes ideas of conflict against an invisible and often mysterious foe is not particularly new.

> However secure and well-regulated civilized life may become, bacteria, Protozoa, viruses, infected fleas, lice, ticks, mosquitoes, bedbugs will always lurk in the shadows ready to pounce when neglect, poverty, famine, or war lets down the defenses. About the only genuine sporting proposition that remains unimpaired by the relentless domestication of a once free-living

human species is the war against these ferocious little fellow creatures, which lurk in the dark corners and stalk us in the bodies of rats, mice, and all kinds of domestic animals; which fly and crawl with insects, and waylay us in our food and drink and even in our love.[6]

These words by Hans Zinsser, written nearly ninety years ago in a book that was praised by the *New York Times* as one of the "wisest and wittiest books that have come off the presses in many a long month," are a reminder that the battle with infection has always scared and fascinated people—even those who were inspired to write because of the mystery of infection. Zinsser was not a novelist but a physician and a bacteriologist.[7] Trained at Columbia University and with a distinguished teaching and research career at Stanford, Columbia, and Harvard, he had a flair for writing. In addition to his academic papers and major discoveries in the lab (the Brill-Zinsser disease is a form of typhoid named after him), he was an extraordinary nonfiction writer and poet.[8] His comfort with the science of bacteriology and his careful reading of history are on full display in his classic text *Rats, Lice and History*, a work still used today to understand the history and impact of typhus fever on human civilization. Zinsser was a pioneer in a long line of writers who brought the knowledge of the laboratory to the public. Some, like Zinsser, Oliver Holmes, and Nawal el Saadawi, and in recent years, Atul Gawande and Siddhartha Mukherjee, have written about their experiences in the lab and the clinic through the medium of essays and creative nonfiction.[9] Others, like Anton Chekhov and Sir Arthur Conan Doyle, brought their medical training to explore ideas around disease like tuberculosis and the life of physicians in everyday life through timeless stories.[10] The physician-writers—often dealing simultaneously with the disease and the lives of the patients—have always brought modern scientific research into the public discourse, challenging our perceptions. Their success has not simply been a result of their extraordinary writing. Many chose infection as the central theme of their writing, and it is the peculiar nature of infection as a disease that draws readers. There is never a shortage of readers who are hungry to learn more about the potential existential threat in their midst.

What does this image of infection have to do with the actual biology of the disease? What is it about the underlying science of infection, the way microbes evolve, live, proliferate, and infect, that causes severe public anxiety and is ripe for political exploitation?

Human experience with infectious diseases goes back to the beginning of our time on this planet.[11] Pathogens—organisms that cause disease in their hosts—predate us by several billion years. Among microbes, bacteria are among the earliest life-forms on the planet, dating back to around 3.5 billion years ago. By comparison, humans have been around for a mere 65 million years. Viruses—microorganisms responsible for a significant number of our infections, including the most recent pandemic—also evolved well before humans. But unlike bacteria, viruses are not considered living organisms as they lack the cellular machinery necessary for independent replication. Viruses are also ten to one hundred times smaller than the smallest bacteria and can only reproduce when they reside inside other organisms, including bacteria.

While a human-centric view of our world may make us believe that pathogens attack or colonize only humans or animals that we interact with, pathogens have been attacking other pathogens before the evolution of humans and animals. The attack-defense-counterattack between microorganisms takes many shapes and forms. For example, viruses can colonize bacteria and commandeer their cellular machinery to fight other bacteria.[12] The battle for resource control and survival has resulted in pathogens fine-tuning their arsenal, picking up a gene or two from other bacteria that gives them an edge, and evolving for efficient survival in harsh environments over the course of millions of years.

Evidence of epidemics and infections goes back millennia.[13] The classical period in Mexico (AD 250–900) marked a period of relative prosperity that came to an end in a devastating population decline in the Terminal Classic period (AD 750–900) that is associated with the spread of disease. In Europe, a millennium and a half before the Black Death (1346–53), there was the Antonine plague (AD 165–90), which peaked during the reign of Roman emperor Marcus Aurelius and had a devastating impact on the empire.[14] Later identified by historians and scientists as potentially a form of smallpox or measles, it quickly spread, decimating the populace.[15] The population decline and loss of manpower resulting from the epidemic most likely weakened the Roman military and the stability and governance of the empire.

A few centuries later, the plague of Justinian (AD 541–49) was the first recorded plague to affect the Mediterranean basin, Europe, and the Near East.[16] According to conservative estimates, the Justinian and Antonine plagues led to the deaths of tens of millions of people. The Justinian pandemic weakened the Byzantine Empire and contributed to the loss of its territory to the Lombards and Goths.

The first confirmed case of the bubonic plague—a bacterial infection spread by infected fleas that leads to, among other things, swollen and painful lymph nodes (called *buboes*)—is documented to have emerged around AD 532 in Egypt and spread through the Middle East in the following years.[17] The second medieval plague pandemic, known commonly as the Black Death, most likely originated in China in 1334 and spread westward along trade routes, reaching Constantinople and eventually Europe, where it killed an estimated 20 to 30 million people, more than a third of the European population.[18] This pandemic, lasting over 130 years, resulted in significant political, economic, cultural, and religious impacts. The Black Death also likely caused a significant labor shortage that contributed to the breakdown of feudalism. This labor shortage also resulted in an expansion in technology adoption in agriculture, which changed Europe's economy and society in the centuries to come.

Another devastating population loss occurred in the sixteenth century, when more than 80 percent of the entire Mesoamerican indigenous population was lost to what is widely believed to be "a series of epidemics of hemorrhagic fever called cocoliztli, a highly lethal disease unknown to both Aztec and European physicians during the colonial era."[19] Francisco Hernández, the *protomédico* of New Spain (that is, a member of the board of physicians in charge of regulating medical practices), witnessed the symptoms of the 1576 cocoliztli infections, describing the fevers as "contagious, burning, and continuous, all of them pestilential, in most part lethal."[20] Hernández also mentioned that the tongues of inflicted individuals were "dry and black" and their urine "the colors sea-green, vegetal-green, and black." Another observer, Dr. Pedro Garcia Farfán, a missionary physician, considered the disease "so dangerous that he recommended that his patients prepare their wills and confess themselves" before they passed. All witnesses mentioned that a striking aspect of this epidemic was its marked selectivity for the indigenous population. Everywhere the disease was reported, the Spanish remained relatively unharmed.

* * * *

THE ORIGIN OF infectious diseases, given the death and destruction that lay in their wake, has always intrigued humans and demanded an explanation—or if not an explanation, a scapegoat, and sometimes both.[21] In the quest to find answers, infection has been blamed on everything from witches to religious and ethnic minorities. Antisemitism was widespread in Europe during the time of the Black Death, and as Jewish people were being blamed for many of the ills that fell on the society, thousands were executed and many more displaced.[22] In a particularly horrific pogrom in Strasbourg, France, on February 14, 1349, as many as several thousand Jewish residents were killed, many of them burned alive, as retribution for the plague.[23]

Repeated instances of various disease outbreaks swept through parts of Europe from the Middle Ages up to the twentieth century. Often, the blame fell on the Jews for spreading the disease. With repeated outbreaks, antisemitic sentiments grew.[24] Pogroms occurred in various cities all across Europe resulting in the killing of thousands of Jewish residents and the forced displacement and expulsion of Jewish populations.

Across the globe, other communities pinned the blame for infections and epidemics on outsiders, typically those deemed an enemy. For example, syphilis—which we now know is a disease caused by the helix-shaped bacterium *Treponema pallidum*—was called the French disease across Europe.[25] The term was first coined by Italians around 1495 as the disease spread in Naples during the French invasion of Italian towns.[26] The association of the French with the syphilis continued for centuries. Even today, searching "French disease" online automatically will direct you to articles about syphilis. Predictably, the French were unhappy with the association, and they came up with their own name: the Neapolitan disease.[27] The blame was not just between the Italians and the French. Other communities had their own culprits.[28] The Russians thought the Poles were responsible, and the Poles called it the German disease. The Danes and the Portuguese called it the Spanish disease. The Turks blamed the Christians, the Hindus of India said the Muslims were responsible, and the Muslims in India said it was the Hindus who had brought the disease to them.[29]

The blame game and speculation about the source of infection often went beyond angry gods, individuals, and communities. When the diseases continued to appear even after retributive killings, expulsions, and exiles, it was hard to find new scapegoats and it was not always possible to pin the blame on outsiders. Some found plausible explanations in the heavens and the astronomical conjunction of the planets and the alignment or misalignment of other heavenly bodies.[30] Others had an even more abstract idea: *air*.[31]

One of the strongest beliefs about the origin of deadly infections, and one that lasted for centuries, was that the disease was in the air. The idea of *miasma*—or bad air—as the cause of infection was first coined in the fourth century BC by Hippocrates and was commonly accepted well into the middle of the nineteenth century.[32] Beyond the ordinary citizens who had faith in this theory, scientists and scholars presented logical arguments in defense of it.[33] The idea of bad air was so deeply rooted that any other possibilities were summarily rejected, even in the presence of objective studies. Though the theory has now been discredited, its legacy continues to this day. The word *malaria*, a mosquito-borne illness caused by a parasite, comes from the merger of two words—*mal* (bad) and *aria* (air).

Interestingly, it was the challenge to the notions of miasma that led to the development of the intellectual tools that are the foundation of modern epidemiology and public health efforts to control infections. The man at the center of the miasma debate was John Snow.[34] Snow was a physician working in London at the time of repeated cholera outbreaks in the city during the middle part of the nineteenth century. Things came to a head in one of the worst outbreaks of cholera in London in 1854. Since the affected communities tended to be known for their foul-smelling air, the idea that cholera was spreading through miasma was hard to refute. Snow had been skeptical of miasma for quite some time and was not convinced of this simple correlation. Instead, based on his prior experience dealing with the outbreaks, he had suspected for some time that contaminated water was the actual source of the infectious disease.

During the 1854 cholera outbreak, he started collecting information on who the patients were, where they were living, and how their houses were getting their water. He was interested in understanding whether there was any link among the people who were falling ill. Through careful investigation and detailed mapping, Snow identified a cluster of cholera cases centered around a water pump on Broad Street (now Broadwick Street). He reviewed his data again and again and concluded that the cause of the outbreak was a contaminated water network that connected everyone who had been ill. He went on to create an illustrated map of the city and where the disease was spreading, supporting his theory with statistical analysis and describing the connection between the quality of the water source and cholera. Not everyone was initially convinced. In time, however, his findings were instrumental in shaping public health policies that prioritized data collection and statistical analyses over dogma and belief. These principles are regarded as the foundations of the modern science of epidemiology.[35]

* * * *

WHAT MAKES INFECTIOUS diseases particularly terrifying is not simply the agony they cause patients and the high likelihood of imminent death from them but their fundamental ability to spread. From one person to another, from one home to the next, the notion that a silent killer can suddenly appear at our doorstep is terrifying. Equally frightening is the idea of our vulnerability to an assault by an unknown and invisible enemy. This lack of immunity—real or perceived—has always had a devastating effect on not just the body but also the psyche of individuals and communities. Not knowing when the disease may attack or how bad it may be can create an immense sense of anxiety, stopping us from acting, or even causing us to give up on life altogether.

Beyond the agony of patients and the anxiety of those who fear the worst, infection also adversely affects livelihoods. The spread of contagion among livestock can lead to starvation. Infectious diseases can cause the collapse of farms large and small.[36] This phenomenon continues in the present as climate change alters the distribution of disease organisms and threatens agriculture in regions all around the globe.[37] Similarly, diseases such as bird and avian flu have had a lasting impact not just on farming communities but also on individuals and institutions directly or peripherally connected to animal and poultry farming.[38] The financial losses in the United States from the 2022 avian flu were estimated to be upward of $2.5 billion.[39]

While some infections are species-specific, plenty of them can jump from one species to another. For example, some infections that find hosts in animals stay with animals and some are able to jump from animals to humans. Diseases that can be transmitted between animals and human are broadly known as *zoonotic diseases*.[40] In some cases, animals act as a reservoir, meaning that the pathogen naturally lives and proliferates in the animal. In other instances, the pathogen may have coevolved and may not cause the disease in the host. But as the pathogen jumps from one species to another, it can become deadly to the newly infected species that may not have the immune system to fight it.

A variety of factors ranging from loss of natural habitat and urbanization to climate change have increased the incidence and spread of zoonotic diseases. Some pathogens also mutate as they move from one species to another, potentially making them more potent over time. Humans, by and large, remain vulnerable to zoonotic infections, as it is exceedingly difficult to know which animal is carrying a disease that can affect humans.

Rabies is among the most well-known examples of a zoonotic disease.[41] The rabies virus affects the central nervous system of mammals, and it is usually transmitted through the bite of an infected animal, commonly bats, dogs, and raccoons. The primary symptoms of rabies are very similar to those of the flu: fever, headache, nausea, vomiting, and agitation. The acute neurologic period begins with signs of central nervous system dysfunction, and symptoms during this stage include agitation, anxiety, hallucinations, and difficulty swallowing. Rabies, though treatable with vaccination, can be fatal if left untreated.[42]

A zoonotic disease does not have to be the result of a direct bite from an infected animal. Plague is one such case.[43] Plague is caused by a bacterium called *Yersinia pestis*, which can be transmitted by infected fleas. These fleas are most often found in small mammals, including rats. As the rodents die, the hungry fleas find other hosts for sources of blood, such as humans. The disease can then spread from one person to the next without an animal as a source or intermediary. The disease can also spread through the inhalation of aerosolized droplets from infected tissues. Plague has three main clinical types. Bubonic plague—the most common of the dreaded disease during Black Death—is marked by lymph node inflammation after a flea bite.[44] Second, the pneumonic plague is transmitted through inhaling droplets from infected humans or animals. Researchers believed that while Black Death was initiated by bubonic plague, it was the pneumonic plague that resulted in the rapid spread from one person to another. The third type is septicemic plague, resulting from the spread of bubonic or pneumonic plague in the bloodstream, and it was the least common during Black Death. It was, however, the most lethal subtype, with near certain mortality of the infected person.

While the incidence of plague has plummeted over the last centuries, other zoonotic diseases have affected millions around the world in recent times.[45] MERS (Middle East Respiratory Syndrome, with camels as the reservoir), Ebola (bats), the Severe Acute Respiratory Syndrome (SARS) outbreak of the early 2000s (bats), Zika (monkeys), and, of course, COVID-19 (also known as SARS-cov-2) are also examples of diseases that can emerge among animals and transmit to humans.[46] The interconnectedness of humans and animals, along with factors such as urbanization, deforestation, and increased global travel, contribute to the potential for zoonotic disease outbreaks. As these diseases spread from one person to another, from one community to the next, they continue to evolve and, at times, become more deadly.

The fear of a novel disease is real. A nation's response to the outbreak of a disease might depend on its economy, particular political realities, and geographic neighborhood. Many countries often respond impulsively. Countries where a disease may have found its first victims worry not just about the disease's impact on their public health but also about its impact on their economy—for instance, from plummeting tourism—and on their international reputation. In trying to protect their image or suppress anxiety among their own citizens, countries often refuse to acknowledge the outbreak or to share data with other nations or international health agencies. Other nations go in a different direction. They will acknowledge the outbreak, but despite weak or no evidence, they are quick to blame entire societies or ethnic communities for the origin of disease.

The origin of a particular infection or outbreak may or may not be obvious, but the ability of an infectious disease to spread among people who come in contact with one another is undeniable. The natural response is to stop the contagion by placing barriers between the infected and the uninfected or by separating the infected from those who might be at risk. The idea of isolating sick patients is not particularly new and has been encouraged in communities throughout history, whether through state decree or religious edict. For example, as part of their religious practice, Muslims in the seventh century were encouraged to stay away from towns affected by the plague, and those who lived in towns that had the plague were told to shelter in place and avoid travel of any kind.[47] Practices such as these laid the basis of modern notions of quarantine.

The idea of quarantine as we know it today probably dates back to the Middle Ages, when it evolved in the port cities of Europe.[48] Diseases are devastating for commerce and trade, especially for towns that are dependent on the movement of people and goods. After repeated bouts of plague, administrators in Italy's coastal cities instituted a practice that would require all incoming ships to sit at anchor for forty days (quarantine comes from medieval Latin word *quarantena*—or forty days) before the passengers and cargo were allowed to disembark.[49] The idea of quarantine was, in part, rooted in the notion that diseases were a result of sin and a divine forty-day period was needed for purification.[50]

While the practice of quarantine had clear success in controlling the rapid spread of the disease in the cities, the impact on those who were confined was not always favorable.[51] The passengers on the quarantined ships often ran out of food and provisions and were at the mercy of the port authorities. In many cases, they died of the combined effects of disease, poor nutrition, and lack of medical care.

* * * *

DESPITE MAJOR SCIENTIFIC advances that argued for quarantine and better hygiene to prevent widespread deaths from infection, it was not until the middle of the nineteenth century that a clear understanding of what causes infection started to emerge. Until then, preventive measures were largely empirical. Understanding about infections was shaped by several theories, including miasma and spontaneous generation. Spontaneous generation was the theory that proposed that living matter (including microbes) could originate from inanimate matter, such as dust, mud, or dead flesh. This idea had been around and accepted by physicians for nearly two millennia, and though some work in the eighteenth century had started to dispute it, it was not until the mid-nineteenth century that the theory was firmly rejected. This change in perspective was not the result of a single development in one discipline but a series of independent discoveries.[52] Through understanding the nature, structure, and function of microbes and the development of better microscopes and imaging, scientists and physicians started to unlock the mysteries of infections and the pathogens that cause them. Alongside new insights into basic biology were new laboratory methods, developed largely in Europe, that helped researchers to isolate microbes and study them systematically.[53]

Building on these scientific discoveries and laboratory technologies, Louis Pasteur in France and Robert Koch in Germany, along with their colleagues, led the development of germ theory.[54] Pasteur and Koch were both brilliant experimentalists. Both worked in the latter half of the nineteenth century and both enjoyed revered public profiles and the extraordinary financial support of the governments in their respective countries. Driven by a nationalist fervor—particularly in the immediate aftermath of the Franco-Prussian War of 1870–71—Pasteur and Koch could not stand each other and went to great lengths to downplay each other's work. Despite this, their work, independently and collectively (though not collaboratively), laid the foundations of modern infectious disease research.

Germ theory is often associated with four postulates as laid out by Koch.[55] These, by and large, have stood the test of time. The first postulate states that microorganisms that cause the ailment must be found in diseased individuals but not in healthy individuals. Second, one should be able to isolate and grow the microorganism from a diseased individual. Third, if a healthy individual is inoculated with the microorganism isolated from a diseased individual, the healthy individual will be infected with the disease. And fourth, the microorganism upon isolation from the inoculated (and diseased) experimental host must be identical to the original microorganism (from the first diseased individual). Germ theory is not a theory about the evolution of germs or their life cycle. That understanding came decades later. Germ theory also does not offer much insight about the structure, size, shape, or function of bacteria. But it does offer a brilliant and reliable way to connect disease with the responsible pathogen.

Like all scientific advancements, Koch's articulation of germ theory was a result of discoveries, theories, and observations made by scientists, physicians and other researchers who came before him. What made Koch's work remarkable was his ability to distill these ideas into a coherent theory despite the relatively simple tools (such as wooden spoons) that were at his disposal to test them. His observations were shaped by his experiences serving in the Franco-Prussian War.[56] During the war, he was stationed in Wöllstein and observed that anthrax was the most common disease among cows in the district. Through a series of careful, repeated experiments, with simple instruments he had fashioned for himself, he identified the bacterium responsible for this disease.

In neighboring France, Pasteur became a national hero for his work on another technology that was to shape the battle against infection permanently—vaccines.[57] Though Edward Jenner, an English physician of the late eighteenth century, had discovered the idea of vaccination, it was Pasteur who pioneered the creation of successful vaccines.[58] In another twist of irony, Pasteur came up with the vaccine for anthrax—the disease that had been the focus of Koch's study across the border.[59]

Germ theory ushered a new systematic study of microbes, or the field of microbiology. While several discoveries about the causes of disease had already been made, the last few decades of the nineteenth century and the early part of the twentieth century are now widely considered the defining age of microbiology. Discoveries, mostly in Europe, during that period led to the identification of microorganisms that are responsible for tuberculosis (TB), syphilis, anthrax, and cholera, just to name a few.[60]

Tuberculosis, called the white death because of the severe paleness of patients, who appeared as if they were being consumed from within, was of particular interest to Koch. His success in identifying the cause of TB further raised his profile as a national and international science hero. It was an old killer, and its origin and the way it spread had long been shrouded in mystery. During the Middle

Ages, a form of the illness (now called Scrofula) was known in England and France as the "king's evil," and it was widely considered to be a hereditary disease that could be healed by a royal touch. On March 24, 1882, Koch isolated and identified the bacterium responsible for tuberculosis and showed that TB was an infectious disease. This discovery was instrumental in understanding the transmission and pathology of tuberculosis and led to advancements in tuberculin skin tests and appropriate treatment.[61]

Cholera was another devastating disease that intrigued researchers and public health officials trying desperately to protect their populations. During the nineteenth century, cholera spread across the world, and it was presumed to have come from the Ganges Delta in India.[62] While John Snow had demonstrated the connection between contaminated water and the transmission of the disease, it was much later, in 1883, when Koch isolated *Vibrio cholerae* during his work in Egypt and India as the specific bacterium responsible for cholera, that the scientific consensus on the cause of the disease really started to change.[63]

The extraordinary progress in microbiology continued with German bacteriologists Fritz Schaudinn and Erich Hoffmann's 1905 discovery of the bacterium *Treponema pallidum* as the causative agent for syphilis.[64] Though this brought an end to the mystery and legends of the origins of syphilis, it did little to cure the racism associated with the disease, whereby it was believed that syphilis manifested itself along racial lines. Less than three decades after Schaudinn and Hoffmann's discovery, U.S. researchers, with the full support of public health authorities, embarked on a research project with Black patients in Alabama that became one of the most prominent medical ethics scandals of the twentieth century.[65]

While Koch and others focused on bacteria and bacterial disease, others found that not all infectious diseases could be traced back to bacteria. Among them was Russian microbiologist Dmitry Ivanovsky, who conducted pioneering research on viral diseases in tobacco plants.[66] Ivanovsky's work led to the first scientific investigations into viruses. In 1892, Ivanovsky observed that the infectious agent responsible for some diseases could pass through a filter that was able to retain and capture bacteria. He concluded that there must be other agents, much smaller than bacteria, that can cause infection. He was dealing with viruses, though he did not call them that.

Building on Ivanovsky's work, Dutch botanist Martinus Beijerinck made significant contributions to the understanding of viruses.[67] In 1898, Beijerinck further investigated the filterable agents and coined the term *virus* to describe them. His work showed that viruses are distinct infectious agents, different from bacteria not just in size but also in unique characteristics not shared by bacteria.

* * * *

THE SCIENTIFIC ADVANCEMENTS in identifying the causes of infections also spurred the natural next question: How to prevent and treat them? Quarantine was a means to stop the spread of infection, but it was not a treatment. Prevention was also an important goal, and there was some hope in the form of a new approach, called *vaccination*, that differed from ingesting herbal or poisonous medicine or engaging in painful bloodletting. Vaccination predates germ theory by several decades. The idea of exposing a small amount of the disease to a patient to protect from a full onslaught of the disease (called *variolation*) had been tried in different parts of the world, including the Ottoman Empire in the sixteenth and seventeenth centuries, where it was attempted against deadly diseases, including smallpox.[68] Building on prior theories and discoveries, an English physician, Sir Edward Jenner, who was familiar with work on inoculation in the Ottoman Empire, developed the first successful vaccine for smallpox, a disease that was responsible for nearly 10 percent of global deaths in his time. Jenner tried something different from what was being practiced then. Instead of exposing the patient to the same disease, as was the practice in variolation, Jenner exposed the patient to a similar but much less lethal disease, in this case, cowpox. In 1796, he carried out his first vaccine trial and showed that exposure with a controlled amount of cowpox may result in the person being unwell for a few days, but it eventually protected them from smallpox. Jenner's work was groundbreaking, and it led to the development of techniques and technologies still used today.[69]

Jenner, Pasteur, and others laid the foundation of modern immunology and the concept of protective immunity.[70] At the individual level, this is understood as the immune system's ability to recognize and defend against specific pathogens, such as viruses and bacteria. On a population scale, it is referred to as *herd immunity*, which signifies indirect protection from infection when a substantial proportion of individuals within that community are immune.

The end of the nineteenth century and the beginning of the twentieth century also saw major developments in the disciplines of pharmacology and chemistry. These disciplines, though distinct from microbiology and bacteriology, had a significant impact on the treatment and prevention of disease. With new discoveries about diseases came the call for better therapeutics. Synthetic drugs, meaning those that are not simply extracted and distilled from natural sources but are made mostly or entirely in the lab, appeared on the market. Given their therapeutic performance, soon there was a great demand for these drugs to be produced in large quantities. New synthesis techniques were developed and better methods of filtration became available to scientists to meet this demand. Paul Ehrlich, a pioneering German scientist and a mentee of Koch's, proposed the idea of a *magic bullet*: a molecule or therapy that can attack the pathogen exclusively, while leaving the host unaffected.[71] This idea was the basis of future research to design better and more effective drugs, including the development of antibiotics.[72]

Advancements in microscopy raised yet another, and perhaps bolder, question: Could a virus be used not as an agent that causes disease but as a tool to fight disease? Since viruses are smaller than bacteria and need a host to survive, scientists wondered if viruses could infect bacteria and commandeer the bacterial machinery, eventually destroying it.[73] The work of a quiet, unassuming British microbiologist, Frederick Twort, and a flamboyant French-Canadian microbiologist, Félix d'Hérelle, opened up the possibility of viruses as a cure for bacterial infections. Phage (from the Greek word meaning to devour) therapy—the idea that a virus can enter the bacterial cell and kill it, just as a chemical drug would—took off in many parts of the world and was the subject of the Pulitzer Prize–winning novel *Arrowsmith* by Sinclair Lewis, published in 1925.[74] Interestingly, the biggest champions of phage therapy were not the affluent research centers in Europe or the United States but the government of the communist Soviet Union. Georgia became a major hub for phage research. Stalin was personally interested in promoting and supporting this research. A research institute in Tbilisi (in Stalin's home region of Georgia) was founded in the early 1920s and became the center of phage therapy research. The institute still stands today.

The interest in phage therapy declined in part because of competition from antibiotics and in part because of prejudice against the Soviets in the United States and Western Europe. Any research coming from the Soviet Union, no matter how good, was to be viewed with suspicion.[75] Today, however, there is renewed interest in phage therapy, including from the U.S. armed forces, as a promising approach against antimicrobial resistance and one that is independent of standard antibiotics.[76] One wonders whether a different approach to research—one that was not clouded by biases—could have resulted in therapies that were available a lot earlier.

The focus on the development of new therapeutics opened up new questions about how to study the evolution of disease in humans and where to find appropriate subjects. From the perspective of European powers, in late 1800s and early 1900s there were plenty of colonial subjects (with no rights and a subhuman status) who could be used for the greater good of humanity.

* * * *

GERM THEORY CREATED a new scientific basis and ushered the birth or development of new disciplines, from immunology to microbiology. Yet old biases and prejudices did not simply disappear overnight. In many ways, over the years, the postulates of germ theory have only strengthened those biases. For example, if the disease were to travel from unhealthy individuals to healthy individuals, could there be individuals and communities that were always sick or unhealthy by virtue of their race or culture or because of poverty? Would interaction with them pose a risk to the fine folk who are healthy? Doesn't the theory then automatically suggest that all resources should be employed to erect barriers between any possible interaction? Should we not isolate those whom the society, and the instruments of the state, deem sick?

Perhaps one of the most ironic aspects of the major advancements in the understanding of infection and infectious diseases is that war has spurred new discoveries and the development of new therapeutics.[77] Events at the battlefront have often resulted in new information about pathogens and diseases, and this argument is sometimes used by those in military sectors as a benefit of "just" wars. The most striking example of this argument is the availability of modern antibiotics following World War II. Antibiotics research and clinical trials were ongoing in England well before the war, but it was the necessity of making them available to all frontline soldiers and producing quality drugs in a short time that prompted the U.S. government and the private sector to fully engaged in the large-scale production of penicillin.[78] These efforts sped the research, discovery, development, and production of more new classes of antibiotics and made them available worldwide. There is no question that antibiotics have saved hundreds of millions of lives worldwide over the last seventy years and continue to do so today, in all parts of the world.

The issue of the long-term, knock-on positive effects of wars on infectious disease research is not particularly straightforward. The issue of intent here is important. The impact on infectious disease understanding, or therapeutic discoveries, is an unintended consequence of the war effort. There is nothing deliberate about these discoveries. There have been many wars that have not led to any new discoveries in infectious diseases. The fact that new discoveries or new drugs came as a result of war is coincidental and cannot justify greater spending on defense or weapons programs. Furthermore, even if we believe that wars have resulted in new discoveries that save hundreds of thousands or millions of lives, the same wars resulted in the deaths of tens of millions. Finally, if the billions of dollars that were spent on the war effort were to be used for research, would that not lead to new discoveries that would save lives without having to kill innocent people?

Fighting disease, whether through prevention or cure, has remained a central feature of human societies. The tools and technologies to accomplish the goal of curing disease and minimizing suffering have continued to evolve. The pathogens, unfortunately, have also been responding to these changes with newer arsenals and mechanisms of their own.[79] Throughout their evolutionary history, both bacteria and viruses have undergone significant genetic changes and adaptations—a process broadly termed as *mutation*. Whether the mutations are random or in response to environmental pressures, they can result in the development of enhanced biological machinery capable of withstanding drugs and changing environments. On our side, the technologies to protect us, to prevent and cure disease, continue to evolve. This tussle between people and pathogens continues to this day, as bacteria and viruses evolve strategies to evade human immune systems and as researchers develop new ways to prevent and treat infectious diseases. What complicates this is not just biological questions about genetic networks and molecular structures but also the question of who gets to benefit from our ingenuity and innovation. Who gets to enjoy the fruits of the labor of this research? We must ask why effective therapies are made available only to a select group of privileged people, while others, who may be equally deserving, are denied those therapies based on race, skin color, national origin, or political prejudice.

3

The Disease and the Outsider

ON JUNE 5, 2020, IN THE ROSE GARDEN OF THE White House, President Donald Trump called the outbreak that came to be known across the world as COVID-19 "the China Plague."[1] This new term had a dual meaning. On the one hand, it was meant to put the responsibility of a seemingly unstoppable disease on China, and on the other, it directly connected this outbreak with a devastating pandemic of the past.

While the term was new, the link between infection and a U.S. administration connecting the origin of the disease with a particular country or community was anything but. In May 1882, 138 years before President Trump made his announcement, another U.S. president, Chester Arthur, signed into law the Chinese Exclusion Act.[2] It was the only act, up until that point, in the history of a country that was nearly a century old, that prohibited migrant laborers from a particular ethnic group, in this case the Chinese, from entering the United States. The Chinese Exclusion Act was the result of decades of discrimination—including the California Supreme Court's 1854 ruling *People v. Hall* that prohibited Chinese people, along with Native American and Black people, from being able to testify against white citizens.[3] Chinese laborers—who were poor and underpaid and often lived in urban slums—were also viewed as immoral and unhygienic. The connection with the spreading of disease was, of course, obvious in the minds of many.[4]

Immigration from China picked up during the California gold rush of 1849, but by 1860, the number of Chinese immigrants in the United States still remained relatively small, at just over 35,000.[5] To put it in context, the total U.S. population in 1860 was well over 31 million, of which Chinese immigrants represented less than 0.15 percent.[6] But Chinese immigration increased following the 1868 Burlingame-Seward Treaty, which allowed for increased bilateral travel and immigration between the United States and China, and by 1880 there were three times as many Chinese immigrants in the United States (approximately 105,000) as there had been in 1860.[7]

A large number of Chinese workers were contracted laborers who were willing to work for lower wages than their white counterparts received in the railroad, garment, and agricultural industries. Because of limited rights, they could not demand higher wages. Moreover, when companies wanted to reduce their spending or replace striking workers, they hired Chinese workers, leading to widespread concern that the Chinese were stealing jobs from white Americans—a feeling that became stronger during the economic downturn of the 1870s. This discontent energized labor leaders like Denis Kearney, who would often end their fiery speeches with such arguments as "And whatever happens, the Chinese must go."[8]

The sentiment about jobs was further boosted by a general belief among white Americans that the Chinese were inferior and fundamentally incapable of assimilating into U.S. society. Justice Stephen J. Field, a U.S. Supreme Court judge, wrote in one of his opinions that Chinese immigrants "have remained among us a separate people, retaining their original peculiarities of dress, manners, habits, and modes of living, which are as marked as their complexion and language. . . . They do not and will not assimilate with our people; and their dying wish is that their bodies may be taken to China for burial."[9] A series of laws in California, driven by xenophobia, were proposed and occasionally passed (though many were vetoed or struck down by courts) that tried to regulate

Chinese cultural practices, such as banning the use of firecrackers and enforcing the Queue Ordinance (in which Chinese prisoners had their hair cut to one inch in length). This perceived fundamental inability of the Chinese to assimilate was combined with anxiety about how the presence of the Chinese (and other East Asian immigrants) would impact the racial makeup of the United States. So while the economy started to improve significantly in the 1880s, the chorus of voices—from workers who believed that the Chinese were taking their jobs and from white Americans who perceived the Chinese as uncivilized and were concerned about the changing demographic and racial makeup of U.S. society—clamoring about the *Chinese Question* continued to rise and became loud enough for President Arthur to sign the Chinese Exclusion Act in 1882.[10]

The new law stipulated a ban on Chinese laborers, "skilled or unskilled," from entry to the United States for ten years.[11] The definition of what accounted for *skilled or unskilled* was left to broad interpretation. And the law was not limited to Chinese who wanted to enter the country for the first time. It also stipulated that Chinese workers who had entered the country before 1882 must get certifications to reenter if they ever chose to leave. Those certifications were almost impossible to obtain. In addition, the U.S. Congress barred federal and state courts from giving citizenship to Chinese residents.

The act had a substantial impact on the entry of Chinese nationals to the United States: between 1880 and 1890, the Chinese population in the United States grew by only 1,852 persons.[12] While there were new laws banning entry of new workers, those already living in the country continued to be deeply affected by discrimination and hate, which sometimes erupted into acts of violence, expulsion, and massacre. Dozens of Chinese miners were killed in 1885 in Wyoming (Rock Springs Massacre) and in 1887 in Oregon (Deep Creek Massacre).[13]

When the Chinese Exclusion Act expired in 1892, Representative Thomas Geary, a Democrat representing California's First Congressional District, sponsored an extension of the original act.[14]

His proposed extension maintained the structure of the original act and added additional clauses. The Geary Act retained the ten-year ban on entry to the United States and also required Chinese laborers within the country to carry an internal passport at all times. Failure to do so meant deportation or hard labor. The new act was challenged as unconstitutional soon after its passage, but the Supreme Court in 1893 rejected the challenge and upheld the act in a 5–3 vote, making it the law of the land.[15]

While the Chinese Exclusion Act was promoted as a necessary step to protect jobs for white Americans, conditions were well suited for a connection with public health to be made and for calls to emerge for the expulsion of Chinese residents from cities, particularly on the West Coast.[16]

In the public imagination, East Asians had long been seen as unhygienic, and Chinatowns were associated with troublesome practices and poor sanitation. Posters published in the 1870s and 1880s connected "vapors" coming from Chinatown in San Francisco with the "Three Graces," namely malaria, smallpox, and leprosy.[17] These posters simultaneously promoted xenophobia and the theory of miasma. Outbreaks of disease in California were often immediately associated with people living in Chinatown and their behavior, regardless of any epidemiological evidence. Writing for the *California History* journal in 1978, Joan Trauner, a medical historian, noted that in the 1870s, the San Francisco Board of Health often characterized health challenges through the lens of politics and social biases, going so far as to "credit Chinatown with introducing and disseminating every epidemic outbreak to hit San Francisco."[18] This despite, as Trauner notes, many on the board not being trained to understand the complex issues of public health. One physician in 1876 expressed frustration about scapegoating the Chinese and wrote that "the Chinese were the focus of Caucasian animosities, and they were made responsible for mishaps in general. A destructive earthquake would probably be charged to their account." Unable to account for the severity of disease outbreaks in San Francisco, the city health officer, J.L. Meares, said, "I unhesitatingly declare my belief that the cause is the presence in our midst of 30,000 (as a class) of unscrupulous, lying and treacherous Chinamen, who have disregarded our sanitary law."[19] This tactic deflected attention from the actual causes of the city's epidemics, which were rooted in the proliferation of infective agents from lack of basic sanitation services.

By framing epidemics as a result of the actions of Chinese residents, Meares attempted to justify even more discriminatory measures. These included segregation, quarantine, and thorough fumigation of every home in Chinatown in 1875 and 1876, as the homes were supposedly dirty and needed to be cleansed. Other forms of social control, such as involuntary confinement, were driven by prejudice rather than by genuine public health concerns.

While the clinical evidence that Chinese people were responsible for disease outbreaks was scant, the support from the public health authorities in blaming them was plentiful. In 1880, the San Francisco Board of Health said that

> the Chinese cancer must be cut out of the heart of our city, root and branch, if we have any regard for its future sanitary welfare . . . with all the vacant and health territory around this city, it is a shame that the very centre be surrendered and abandoned to this health-defying and law-defying population. We, therefore, recommend that the portion of the city here described be condemned as a nuisance; and we call upon the proper authorities to take the necessary steps for its abatement without delay.[20]

Another health official considered Chinatown a moral purgatory in the city "through which all who pass come out nauseated and disgusted and perchance defiled by Mongolian filth or disease."[21]

* * * *

THE XENOPHOBIA AGAINST Chinese people was fueled by a flawed, or perhaps deliberately disingenuous, understanding of a whole host of infectious diseases. High on this list of diseases that stigmatized the poor and the foreigner was leprosy.[22] Patients suffering leprosy were often viewed as immoral and ugly. Their suffering and deteriorating appearance were blamed on their sinful behavior. This association between personal and moral failings and disease merged seamlessly with widespread xenophobia in the society around the turn of the century, particularly in San Francisco. The bacterium that causes leprosy was discovered by Gerhard-Henrik Armaeur Hansen in 1873, but the myth surrounding the disease's origin and spread remained a part of the public psyche for decades to follow.[23] One San Francisco health official believed that leprosy among the Chinese was "simply the result of generations of syphilis, transmitted from one generation to another."[24] Dr. Joseph Jones, the former head of the Louisiana Board of Health, said that Chinese laundrymen working in San Francisco, Louisiana, and New York were "in the early stages of the disease; and their practice of taking water in their mouths and spitting it out on the clothes they iron, is more than ever disgusting when considered in connection with the possible transmission of disease by this means."[25] Furthermore, he added that the United States would see widespread leprosy because of the "filthy . . . unprincipled, vicious, and leprous hordes of Asia." The disease among the Asians came to be known as "Asiatic" or "Oriental" leprosy, which was biologically and clinically identical to the disease seen in native-born white people in the United States and among those Norwegians who brought the disease from Scandinavia to the Upper Midwest.[26] As a result of xenophobia, leprosy patients from Chinatown in San Francisco were rounded up and sent back to China at the first opportunity. Chinatown, as one historian has noted, was considered a laboratory of infection.[27]

Numerous attempts were made from the late nineteenth through early twentieth centuries to either completely depopulate

San Francisco's Chinatown or relocate its residents far outside the city. When neither of those options proved viable, proposals were made by the local officials to ensure that no real support or health care access was provided to the residents of Chinatown.

During the nineteenth century and the early part of the twentieth century, the issues of public health, and by extension infection, became intertwined with immigration policy, acceptance of immigrants, and perceptions about their integration into U.S. society. Between 1820 and 1924, approximately 36 million people immigrated to the United States, with the East Coast receiving many immigrants from Eastern, Central, and Southern Europe; the West Coast, accepting arrivals from Japan, China, and Mongolia; and the southern border, those from Mexico.[28] A relatively small number of immigrants came across the northern border with Canada. As the number of arrivals increased (particularly via Ellis Island in New York), a distinction was made between the old immigrant and the new. The old immigrants were those who came from Northern Europe, namely Great Britain, Scotland, Ireland, Germany, France, and the Scandinavian countries. In contrast, the inflow of immigrants during the nineteenth and early twentieths centuries largely came from eastern and southern Europe, including Russia, Greece, Italy, Spain, the Austro-Hungarian Empire, and the Balkans. These new immigrants—among them Eastern Europeans and Jews—were viewed as dirty, uneducated, and unlikely to assimilate into American society.[29] They were also viewed as people who were likely to bring disease to American shores. During this period, ideas of evolution and the inherent superiority and inferiority of various races were widely supported and used to proclaim the new immigrants as biologically inferior on the basis of their race, and were described as "swarthy, squalid, pestilent or of bad stock."[30]

For those who came on ships, poor sanitation, lack of food, and cramped compartments meant the high likelihood of disease spread. The presence of disease on these ships resulted in U.S. policies forcing all steamships to inspect and "disinfect" all immigrants before departure from foreign shores.[31] Some immigrants who underwent tests and observation at the port of entry were turned back or detained for weeks, months, or more at U.S. Public Health Service hospitals. Inspection and observation at the arrival centers, unsurprisingly, followed the social perceptions of the time. People from Mexico and China were treated harshly and scrutinized far more than white immigrants from Northern Europe. They were more frequently poked for blood samples and treated with harsh chemical agents as disinfectants.[32] Eye exams for trachoma (a bacterial infection) were particularly horrific.[33] At the same time, far more immigrants on the West Coast were debarred or deported than were those on Ellis Island, suggesting a strong racial and xenophobic attitude toward nonwhite immigrants.[34] Research suggests that between 1890 and 1924, approximately 15 million new immigrants, mostly from Europe, arrived at Ellis Island. Out of these, approximately only 1 percent were turned back. In contrast, at Angel Island (in San Francisco), between 1910 and 1940, 17 percent of immigrants from China, Japan, and Korea were debarred.[35] There was also a marked difference between those who walked across from the northern border (Canada) and those came from the south (Mexico). While there were some minor concerns about those of French descent and their ability to fully integrate into American society (compared with British immigrants, whose assimilation was never questioned), such xenophobic alarms were much louder regarding immigrants crossing the southern border.[36]

During the last decades of the nineteenth century, disease outbreaks were viewed not simply as a public health issue but also as an issue of economic stability. Immigration, disease, and economy often wound up in a continuum of policy discussions. While treatment options were still somewhat ad hoc and not always effective, it had been established that hygiene and sanitation are critical for the effective control of infection, particularly waterborne diseases. During this period, the state health laboratories were established, the first one in Massachusetts in the 1890s.[37] Similarly, quarantine, as noted in the previous chapter, had been established as a viable strategy to control epidemics, though its application was greatly influenced by political views and racial prejudices. Up until this point, quarantines were managed by individual states, but that was soon to change.

On February 15, 1893, Congress passed the National Quarantine Act, or more formally, "An Act Granting Additional Quarantine Powers and Imposing Additional Duties upon the Marine-Hospital Service."[38] This act gave the federal government the right to create a national system of quarantine, while also maintaining state-run quarantines. The act also authorized the president of the United States to "prohibit, in whole or in part, the introduction of persons and property from such countries or places as he shall designate for such period of time as he may deem necessary."[39] For a period of nearly thirty years, the act was used by the federal and state governments to control the spread of diseases, including cholera, smallpox, yellow fever, and other infectious outbreaks of concern.

Quarantine measures were often intertwined with prevailing xenophobia and public opinion that dictated public health policies in the country at that time. In 1900, when an autopsy of a Chinese man suggested that his body had been colonized by plague-causing bacteria, the city of San Francisco restricted the movement of *all* Chinese residents.[40] They, and only they, were prohibited from leaving the city. Similar instances targeted Mexican immigrants in Texas. In 1915, Mexico was hit hard by a typhus outbreak during its revolutionary war.[41] Poor sanitation, poverty, and overcrowding contributed to several Mexican cities experiencing a deadly wave of the disease. In late 1916, several cases of typhus fever were noticed north of the U.S.-Mexico border in El Paso, Texas. The U.S. Public Health Service (PHS) responded with an aggressive and large-scale quarantine program. The PHS physician in charge of the quarantine wrote that the goal of the quarantine campaign was to disinfect anyone who was "considered as likely to be vermin infested."[42] People in the quarantine were inhumanely treated. They were stripped naked in front of attending public health workers and examined for lice and nits and doused with kerosine. They were then given a certificate from PHS verifying that the person had been "deloused, bathed, vaccinated, clothing and baggage disinfected."[43] The quarantine and inspection protocol stayed in place until the 1930s, well after the typhus epidemic had ended. The aggressive strategy was selectively applied along socioeconomic lines and visible signs of wealth and affluence. Those traveling across the southern border in first-class cabins on trains or who were well dressed were exempted from these harsh measures. While the quarantine measures are no longer in place, historians Markel and Stern note that these measures have had a lasting impact on the public psyche, suggesting that the "harsh reality and duration of the quarantine helped generate and underscore stereotypes of Mexicans as impure and infectious."[44] Some of these perceptions that became particularly prominent during the pandemic were amplified by public officials in the southern states.[45]

* * * *

IN THE LAST decade of the nineteenth century and the first quarter of the twentieth, the quarantine law of 1893 was used (and abused) against people already present in the country and those who had already arrived at U.S. ports of entry. The law, up until that point, had not been used to refuse entry to the country. This changed in 1929.

The election on November 6, 1928, resulted in a landslide victory for the Republican candidate, Herbert Hoover.[46] By the time he was inaugurated in January 1929, there had been repeated outbreaks of meningitis (an infection that results in inflammation of the tissue around the brain and the spinal cord) all across the country, including the Northeast, the Midwest, and along the Pacific Coast.[47] The number of cases had been steadily rising over the previous two years. During that same period, there were frequent reports of meningitis in East Asia, including China, Japan, and the Philippines.[48] Without much research or evidence, authorities linked the outbreak in the United States to the passengers and vessels coming from East Asia, in particular China and the Philippines. While the disease patterns (rise and fall, number of cases, etc.) in the U.S. mirrored what was going on in Europe, particularly in England and Wales, the immigration patterns in the United States and Europe were quite dissimilar. The argument that it was largely people arriving from Asia, China in particular, who were responsible for the outbreaks in the U.S. did not quite hold up, since there was comparatively little immigration of the Chinese to Europe, yet the disease patterns were similar. The Hoover administration, in its early years, wanted to appear strong and felt that it needed to act decisively. On June 21, 1929, President Hoover issued an order that restricted the arrival of all ships from China and the Philippines.[49] By that time, the number of Chinese immigrants had already decreased substantially because of the Exclusion and Geary Acts, dropping from 107,000 in 1890 to about 61,000 in 1920.[50] A further decline occurred following the Immigration Act of 1924 (also known as the National Origins Act), which imposed strict quotas on immigrants entering the United States and debarred all Asian immigrants from the possibility of naturalization.[51] Fear of germs and diseases and a perception that certain races are inferior and hence prone to disease and likely to spread those diseases to local populations empowered the nativist groups in successfully passing the act, which stayed in place until 1964.

Despite the exclusion acts of the previous century, several thousand Chinese immigrants from 1910 onward were able to satisfy the authorities at Angel Island (San Francisco) and enter the country legally to meet the growing demand of workers in the country.[52] President Hoover's new order, however, was going to make things more complicated for Chinese immigrants (along with others coming from Asia). The statement codifying the new decree said that "it is ordered that no persons may be introduced directly or indirectly by transshipment or otherwise into the United States or any of its possessions or dependencies from any port in China (including Hong Kong) or the Philippine Islands for such period of time as may be deemed necessary, except under such conditions as may be prescribed by the Secretary of the Treasury."[53]

The order was made public by the State Department on July 8 and appeared in newspapers around the country the following day. To give his order legal cover, Hoover used the 1893 quarantine act to restrict the entrance of *all* persons from China and the Philippines for as long as necessary.

This was the first time people from specific countries were refused entry for reasons of public health. The prior acts were based on an interconnected set of reasons that included jobs and the labor market and perceptions about integration and assimilation in the U.S. The Hoover decree was different because it argued that vessels coming from China and the Philippines could bring disease that would put American lives at risk. More important was the fact that this decree went beyond individuals (as was the case on Ellis Island) or vessels that had sick passengers. This was a blanket decree—based on weak epidemiology and strong racial motives.

In its defense, the government did not claim that there were strong moral or clinical reasons for this order. Instead, it claimed that the government had limited available facilities at its disposal and that the few existing facilities were already stretched thin and hence unable to deal with an influx of new patients and likely outbreaks. The order made this point clear, stating, "whereas the continued arrival of vessels having epidemic cerebrospinal meningitis infection on board has overtaxed the combined available quarantine facilities of federal and local health authorities and that notwithstanding the quarantine defense, there exists danger of introducing this disease into the United States."[54]

The argument was that establishing and staffing more quarantine centers was not possible because of limited resources. Without quarantine centers, the disease could spread throughout the country. It just happened to be a mere coincidence that the citizens barred from coming were members of racial and ethnic communities that evoked racist and xenophobic sentiments among sections of the U.S. population.

The executive order signed by President Hoover was built on the premise that the number of meningitis cases would continue to increase, particularly on the West Coast. This was not backed up by epidemiological data available at the time. A careful examination of the records in the years prior to the signing of the act suggests that there was no reason to expect a major outbreak or spike. For example, in 1927, there were 260 cases and 101 deaths from meningitis in California. In 1928, there were 259 cases and 115 deaths. By mid-1929, when the executive order was signed into law, there had been a total of 695 cases and 381 deaths. Out of the 381 deaths, 57 were Filipino, 39 were Mexican, 16 were Chinese, and 6 were Japanese.[55] A possible explanation for the deaths among immigrants could be the difficult conditions in which they lived and worked and the limited access to health care available to nonwhite immigrants. However, this was never seriously considered. An increase in the number of cases was also seen in Washington State in 1929 compared with previous years.[56] It was easy to conclude that the disease was coming from the ports of the Philippines and China, but something was amiss. The meningitis epidemic had already been underway in states not on the West Coast for a number of years before the spike in California and Washington occurred. In fact, these outbreaks in other states (far from the ports where the vessels from China and the Philippines were coming) were far more acute. The Weekly Epidemiological Record of the Health Section of the League of Nations noted that

> the epidemic in the United States did not begin on the Pacific Coast but in the Rocky Mountain states and in the City of New York. Thus, in 1928, there were serious epidemics in Montana,

Wyoming, Colorado and Arizona. The maximum came earlier
in New York City than in California, also in 1929. The state
that suffered most severely was Michigan, where 1876 cases
were reported in 1929. In New York City, there were 986 cases
in 1929.[57]

Those in favor of the blanket ban on the arrival of immigrants
from Asia also assumed that the meningitis outbreak in the Pacific
states was due to a type of strain that was unique to the Philippines.
This was also not true. Researchers found that the types of strains
present in the Philippines (and likely to be among those in the vessels departing the country) were not the ones infecting Filipino immigrants in the United States. There was no link between the
disease in Asia and what was seen among the Asian immigrants in
the United States. The senior surgeon of the U.S. Public Health
Service, J.C. Perry, concluded: "I believe that the high incidence of
meningitis in the Pacific Coast and adjoining states was independent
of the prevalence of the disease in the Orient and the infection on
arriving vessels. It was a cumulative effect from preceding years, as
occurs in the cyclical development of outbreaks of meningitis. In
various parts of the United States and other countries, 1929 was a
meningitis year. It has been shown that the Filipinos played no part
in serious outbreaks in two adjoining states. No case was reported
among the Filipinos in San Francisco in 1928, and it was not until
February 1929, that cases of meningitis commenced to appear
among them."[58] He further noted that "the arrivals of Filipinos
and Chinese from infected ports and on ships with disease on board
cannot be held responsible for the outbreak of meningitis in Pacific
Coast States."[59] The report by Dr. Perry—however—did say that
it was most likely the abject poverty and miserable conditions in the
city where the immigrants are forced to live (and not on the ports
from which they embarked) that can lead to disease outbreaks.
"These people crowd together in boarding houses or small flats
for economic reasons, and consequently favorable conditions are

created for the development of the disease among them," he wrote toward the end of his report.

In the midst of the turmoil of the 1929 stock market crash and the resulting Great Depression, the Hoover administration's prohibition on ships coming from parts of Asia to enter the United States was no longer on the minds of the public. The economic conditions in the United States, along with the lasting effects of the 1924 National Origins Act, was reshaping U.S. society and its racial makeup. The 1929 proclamation was the only time the 1893 Quarantine Act was used to close borders to a group of people and deny entry to an individual or a group of individuals, using the potential for a disease outbreak in the country as the main reason. Despite the attention moving elsewhere and the realities of the Great Depression and, later, the horrors of World War II, the law was still on the books and available to be exploited for political expediencies. Fifteen years after the 1929 proclamation, the legal foundations were used to create a new law with a peculiar name: Title 42.

4

Importing and Exporting Cholera

With the danger of cholera in question, it is plain to see that the United States would be better off if ignorant Russian Jews and Hungarians were denied refuge here. These people are offensive enough at best; under the present circumstances they are a positive menace to the health of this country. Even should they pass the quarantine officials, their mode of life when they settle down makes them always a source of danger. Cholera, it must be remembered, originates in the homes of human riffraff.

New York Times, August 29, 1892

CHOLERA IS CAUSED BY A CURVED BACTERIUM that, under the microscope, can look like a large comma.[1] Other images of the bacterium show a rod-like structure connected to a thin tail, known as the *flagellum*. This flagellum (plural *flagella*) serves as a tiny but powerful propeller that allows the bacterium to move, turn, twist, and reach new environments.[2] This characteristic of the bacterium that causes cholera to move is reflected in its formal name: *Vibrio cholerae*; the word *vibrio* meaning "agility," or the ability to move.

The first known cholera epidemic originated in the Ganges Delta in northeast India in 1817 and spread to other parts of Asia.[3] Common symptoms include severe vomiting and watery diarrhea, much like many other ailments of the stomach or intestine. As a result, it has not always been easy to separate cholera from other similar, but perhaps less deadly diseases. Once inside the gut, cholera bacteria divide rapidly and start to colonize the small intestine, typically twelve to seventy-two hours before symptoms appear.[4] Unfortunately, once the symptoms appear, the decline in the patient's health is often rapid. Acute watery diarrhea alone can result in the loss of as much as one liter of fluid per hour.[5] The patient loses essential metabolites and ions and becomes dehydrated, causing severe cramps and leading to collapse of the circulatory system.

The watery stool of a person with cholera can have as many as trillions of vibrio bacteria per liter.[6] In places lacking proper sanitation, contamination of water by infected stool results in the rapid spread of the disease across households and communities.[7]

While humans had suffered from cholera for a long time, it was not until the middle of the nineteenth century that the cause of the disease was finally isolated. The cholera-causing bacterium was first discovered by an Italian professor of anatomy, Filippo Pacini, in Florence in 1854.[8] That year, Europe was in the midst of yet another terrifying cholera outbreak. Coincidentally, this was the same year that the English physician John Snow studied the cholera outbreak in London and showed how poor sanitation conditions in the city contributed to its spread. Snow, much to the dismay of local authorities, had identified a fecal-to-oral route.[9] In doing so, he laid the foundation of modern epidemiology—the science of how and why diseases spread in various communities.[10]

Across the European continent, Pacini worked with the corpses of patients who had recently died of cholera in the public hospital of Santa Maria Nuova in Florence.[11] He also examined the corpses of the washerwomen who were in charge of cleaning the hospital linen and had recently died as well. During his autopsy of the stomach and the intestine, Pacini saw millions of comma-shaped bacteria, which he named *vibrios*. Arguing against the mythical bad air (miasma) hypothesis that was assumed to be the cause of disease at the time but could not be seen or proven through scientific methods, he wrote that the vibrio "exists, can be seen, and it's not presumed."[12] He referred to vibrio as a real element of infection, an "organic, living substance, of parasitic nature, communicating, reproducing, and then producing a disease of special character."

Despite a clear causative agent and strong clinical evidence to support his finding, Pacini found very few supporters for his discovery among the clinical research community. Miasma continued to be the accepted cause. The miasma camp was led by a prominent German scientist, Max von Pettenkofer, who argued that cholera was in fact an airborne disease that was caused by a combination of bad air, seasonal variations, and an innate predisposition to disease.[13] No wonder, according to this camp, that cholera was often present in places with a foul smell.

It took another three decades for the bacterial origin theory of cholera to gain more scientific traction. This time, the lead researcher was someone with immense fame and a large following who could not be dismissed so easily: Robert Koch. Working first in Egypt during a cholera outbreak of 1883 and then in India, Koch used solid surfaces (including potato slices) instead of a liquid medium to isolate and culture the bacteria from the intestines of deceased patients.[14] In Egypt, Koch and his colleagues observed that only the patients who had died of cholera had the particular bacteria in their guts. He was, at that time, unsure whether the bacteria were the cause or if their presence was simply a correlation. This was to change during his work in Calcutta in the later part of the year.[15] He noted that the bacteria were bent, like a comma, which was different from other bacteria seen in other diseases. On January 7, 1884, Koch announced his big discovery and followed it up with evidence in a series of dispatches back to Berlin. Koch, like Snow and Pacini, also argued for clean water and hygiene to prevent the spread of the disease.[16] Even with Koch's fame and reputation, and strong evidence, many still remained unconvinced for years to come. Over time and with mounting evidence from across the world, Pacini's and Koch's discoveries prevailed—though the final piece of the cholera puzzle did not come until 1959, when the toxin for the disease was discovered.[17]

* * * *

BY THE TIME the cover story in the *New York Times* appeared in 1892, with the title "No Way to Stop Immigration: Quarantine the Only Safeguard Against Cholera" the bacterial origin of cholera and the works of Koch, Snow, and others were well known. The information had been reported in scientific journals, which were available to scientists and clinicians working in the United States. The claim that the disease originated in the homes of "riffraff" was no longer an issue of major scientific debate. A careful journalist would have been able to review the scientific information and deduce that simple person-to-person contact did not spread the disease. But cholera, like many other infectious diseases, provided ripe opportunities to oppress and control the lives of undesirables among a community. As a result, despite all of the scientific evidence proving otherwise, public perception continued to connect cholera to Hungarians, Russians, and other immigrant communities.

The Irish, for example, were a regular target of prejudice in the United States during the middle of the nineteenth century. Approximately 2 million Irish refugees sought solace in the United States from the potato famine in Ireland. They were often blamed for diseases, including cholera, that plagued them during their journey across the Atlantic in overcrowded cargo ships with minimal sanitation. The death rate was so high on these ships that these vessels were named *coffin ships*.[18] Tragically, the blame for the afflictions was put not on the conditions but on the Irish passengers and their inherent predisposition to disease.[19]

The Irish who made it to America often found themselves relegated to labor-intensive and hazardous occupations, for which they received inadequate wages. They toiled constructing canals, digging trenches for water and sewer systems, laying railway tracks, cleaning houses, and working in textile mills. In these environments, with poor sanitation, cholera outbreaks emerged frequently.[20] They also often crowded into subdivided homes that were intended for single families. Cellars, attics, and make-do spaces in alleys became home. As the Library of Congress document on assimilation notes, "a lack of adequate sewage and running water in these places made cleanliness next to impossible. Disease of all kinds (including cholera, typhus, tuberculosis, and mental illness) resulted from these miserable living conditions. Irish immigrants sometimes faced hostility from other groups in the U.S., and were accused of spreading disease and blamed for the unsanitary conditions many lived in."[21]

The United States reached epidemic levels of cholera several times during the mid-nineteenth century, particularly during 1832, 1849, and 1866, and Irish communities were impacted frequently by the disease.[22] Digitized Cincinnati birth and death records show that 422 Irish immigrants died from cholera between 1865 and 1912.[23] In addition to xenophobia and anti-poor sentiment, Irish immigrants also experienced religious bigotry, and some nativist Protestant groups viewed cholera as a sign of punishment for the sinful behavior of Catholics. As Walter Daly notes, "It was not uncommon for cholera to be blamed on the Irish due to their religion (anti-Catholic sentiments blamed the disease on a vengeful God) or because of their poor living conditions."[24]

The public perception connecting cholera and the "uncivilized" and unwelcomed immigrants continued for decades, well after the wave of Irish immigration had subsided.

* * * *

THE STORY OF cholera and its relationship with politics and policies did not end with Koch's germ theory, the discovery of the comma-shaped pathogen, or new developments in the science of infectious disease at the turn of the nineteenth century. While cholera may be caused by bacteria, and we now know the molecular structure of the toxin well, it is our collective apathy toward the weak, vulnerable, and poor that is allowing this preventable disease to continue to wreak havoc in communities. Today, cholera is rarely a problem in high-income countries, but outbreaks in poor countries are not unusual.[25]

Additionally, cholera outbreaks often correlate with armed conflicts. In the twenty-first century, cholera has frequently emerged in impoverished communities on the receiving end of aggressive onslaughts made possible by weapons of ever-greater firepower—gladly supplied by countries with large weapons manufacturing capacity.[26]

Yemen, a country that has faced violent conflict fueled by weapons sold by rich countries, has seen repeated, and devastating, outbreaks of cholera in the last decade.[27] Cholera in Yemen is driven not simply by decades of neglect, a weak health system, and abject poverty but also by the deliberate and sustained destruction of urban infrastructure, including hospitals and water supply and sanitation systems.[28] Hospitals and health care centers in Yemen were repeatedly targeted during the conflict, resulting not only in direct casualties and denial of care to those who were sick but also in the spread of infection in the community. The lack of accountability for the cholera outbreak in Yemen is also a matter of concern. Despite the scale of the epidemic, which reached, at its peak, over a million infections and thousands of deaths, no individuals or entities have ever been held responsible for the situation.[29]

Humanitarian organizations have worked tirelessly to provide medical care, clean water, vaccinations, and sanitation services to affected communities, but they are often unable to deliver this help because of limited funds.[30] Additionally, these efforts are often insufficient as there is widespread agreement among public health researchers that the prevention and control of cholera should focus not only on immediate medical interventions but also on addressing the root causes, including the provision of clean water, sanitation facilities, and adequate health care services.[31] Such prevention measures become impossible during an armed conflict with frequent use of heavy weapons.

The complete negligence for the concerns of a poor country, by the states that are eager to sell weapons, and the disregard for the lives of the inconsequential inhabitants of the country on the receiving end of those weapons, allow the cholera epidemics to continue unabated. Despite creating one of the worst cholera outbreaks the world has seen in the last several decades, the existing global system of indifference for the concerns of the poor means that no one can, or will be, held accountable.

Situations like these are often dismissed as the consequences of war, but they are in fact more than that. As researchers and public health workers on the ground have pointed out, the new face of cholera is not simply a natural outcome of poverty but a creation of armed conflict.[32] The Yemen country director of Save the Children was clear in his assessment when he said that "there's no doubt this is a man-made crisis."[33]

The man-made crisis was made possible by weapons sold largely by the United States and the West.[34] Efforts to stop the sale of weapons—which were directly responsible for creating unmitigated outbreaks of cholera among noncombatant Yemenis—did not get much traction. A bipartisan effort by lawmakers to stop the sale of weapons to Saudi Arabia was vetoed by President Donald Trump in 2019, who argued that while endless wars were not the answer, the situation in Yemen was "different."[35] During the Biden administration, the weapons sales to Saudi Arabia were stopped, only to be resumed again in the summer of 2024, while President Biden was still in office.[36]

Whereas the interest in selling weapons is long-standing, the appetite for giving aid that can save lives is often fleeting and temporary. With new conflicts (for example, Ukraine and Israel/Palestine) grabbing the attention of rich countries, the long-term aid that is needed to rebuild the infrastructure and create robust public health structures in Yemen has now all but disappeared. It was inadequate to begin with, even during the height of the crisis when international donors were providing less than 40 percent of the funds needed to keep the barest of operations running.[37] But even that support has now evaporated. The Russian-led war in Ukraine diverted attention and resources away from Yemen and its health care needs. It also diverted media attention and news about Yemen's dilapidated hospitals and continued challenges with clean water. At the time of this writing, the conflict in Yemen has come down from its height of the last decade, and there has been much-needed discussion on peace from all sides, but the health infrastructure remains just as precarious and the humanitarian crisis just as acute. In May 2024, the UN and its agencies reported yet another escalation of cholera in the country, with nearly 30,000 cases between January and April of that year.[38] In the absence of real attention, resources, and training (none of which are happening right now), another major outbreak that could cause widespread mortality and morbidity is lurking just underneath the surface. Weapons made in countries far from the conflict—and sold to some of the richest countries in the region—have created a near permanent epidemic among some of the poorest people on the planet.

Cholera is, unfortunately, just one example of a disease outbreak caused by conflict. The emergence of drug-resistant pathogens as a result of using weapons with heavy metals is another.[39] This consequence is often long-ranging and intergenerational, affecting individuals who are born years after the conflict.

* * * *

BEYOND CONFLICT, THE story of cholera impacting poor countries has unfolded in other disturbing ways. Haiti, a country that despite being among the poorest in the world, had never had a cholera outbreak in its entire history until foreign troops brought it there.[40]

The story of cholera's arrival in Haiti started in the aftermath of a devastating 7.0 magnitude earthquake on January 12, 2010, that occurred approximately 25 kilometers southwest of the Haitian capital of Port-au-Prince. As many as 222,570 people were killed and 300,000 left injured, some with permanent life-changing disabilities.[41] Another 1.3 million, approximately 10 percent of the entire population, were displaced.[42] More than 97,000 houses were destroyed completely and over 180,000 houses were badly damaged, many beyond any chance of repair.[43] The earthquake damaged not just houses and dwellings but major buildings, including the UN headquarters in Port-au-Prince, which collapsed as a result of the earthquake, killing the UN country head, Hédi Annabi.[44]

Pledges of international aid were made to a country that had limited local capacity to distribute it in an organized manner and get it to the areas most affected by the tragedy. Public order started to break down as food and lifesaving supplies dwindled. UN peacekeepers were brought in (in addition to those who were already stationed in the country as part of a previous UN mission that had been in the country since 2004) both to rebuild the infrastructure and to ensure public order.[45]

Nine months after the earthquake, in October 2010, a group of peacekeepers arrived from Nepal.[46] The UN mission stationed them at an outpost in the town of Meye, which is approximately 40 kilometers northeast of Port-au-Prince. That outpost is very close to a tributary of the Artibonite River, the main river in the country, which provides water for drinking, cooking, cleaning, and bathing to a large number of Haitians.[47] These UN peacekeepers had been previously stationed in a place in Nepal that had been experiencing a cholera outbreak.[48] Cholera is also endemic to Nepal and outbreaks there are not unheard of.[49] By the time the Nepalese contingent arrived in Haiti, some of the peacekeepers were already sick with cholera (though probably not showing any serious symptoms). But none of them were tested, according to the testimony of Brigadier General Dr. Kishore Rana, the Nepalese army's chief medical officer.[50] Such testing would have cost less than three dollars per peacekeeper, an insignificant sum when viewed in light of the UN's budget and expenditures.[51] The UN did not require such testing unless a soldier displayed cholera symptoms.[52]

The makeshift UN facilities where the Nepalese peacekeepers were stationed were poorly constructed.[53] Soon after the arrival of the peacekeepers, one of the sewage reservoirs in their housing camp leaked, spreading cholera-infected wastewater to the waterways.[54] As the local residents came in contact with the contaminated water—drank it, used it for washing, and cooked with it—they started getting sick.

Because of the high infectivity of the disease, the number of cases started to rise quickly. Within the first month of the epidemic, nearly 2,000 people died.[55] By July 2011, a person was infected every minute and, as one report noted later, "the total number of Haitians infected with cholera surpassed the combined infected population of the rest of the world."[56] Despite the massive outbreak, the age-old ideas about blaming the poor for their disease went into full swing. It was assumed by international agencies, including the UN, that since the Haitians were poor and lacked good sanitation facilities, cholera was inevitable.[57] Scientific evidence, however, said otherwise. The cholera strains isolated in Haiti were found to be a perfect match with the strains in Nepal. A team of researchers from Haiti, France, and the United States with expertise in public health, genomics and epidemiology was clear in its assessment: "All of the scientific evidence shows that cholera was brought by a contingent of soldiers travelling from a country experiencing a cholera epidemic. Understanding what triggered the epidemic is important for preventing future occurrences, and acknowledges the right of Haitians to understand the events that led to their cholera devastation."[58]

* * * *

DESPITE UNDENIABLE EVIDENCE linking the source of the cholera outbreak and the fact that cholera was not native to

Haiti, the UN flatly denied any responsibility. Parallel to this denial, the cholera outbreak that had started in a UN camp ravaged the country at an astronomical rate. It soon became a permanent feature of the public health challenges faced by Haitians. The locals, who were mostly poor, struggling to make ends meet, undernourished, and displaced, started to fall sick by a disease they had not seen before.[59] There was no prior knowledge of the disease and no local history of how to manage this alien calamity.

The UN peacekeepers in Haiti did not have a great record to begin with. There were already reports of human rights abuses by UN peacekeepers in Haiti, including instances of rape, sexual abuse, and physical assault.[60] With the cholera outbreak, and its connection with the outpost managed by the UN, the locals became increasingly anxious, angry, and deeply suspicious of the UN.

Within a few years, almost ten thousand people had died and over half a million became sick.[61] Researchers believe that these numbers are probably an underestimate because of poor reporting structures and lack of coordination between health centers in the country.[62] Mortality and morbidity due to cholera was in addition to the trauma, injuries, and illnesses that were a result of the earthquake and painfully slow rebuilding. In a poverty-stricken country, the impact on individuals and whole families was devastating. Many of the people who died were the main breadwinners for their families.[63] Their deaths pushed their families further into abject poverty.

The cholera tragedy continued without many answers or any responsibility from the UN and its various offices in the country. Haitians got only vague answers and denial in high doses from the global organization with a mandate to protect people and uphold the highest principles of humanity and human rights.[64]

Within a couple of years of the outbreak, irrefutable epidemiological evidence linked the epidemic with the troops coming from Nepal and the fecal contamination of waterways by the UN peacekeepers. Despite this genomic and epidemiological evidence, the

UN offices in Haiti and its headquarters in New York were unwilling to accept responsibility. Instead, they continued to push back.[65] In 2011, when Haitian and a U.S.-based human rights organizations filed a complaint with the UN on behalf of several thousand victims and demanded reparations, the UN refused to respond for a year, and then in February 2013 it dismissed the claims altogether, invoking clauses of the Convention on Privileges and Immunities of the United Nations.[66] UN Secretary General Ban Ki-moon called Haitian president Michel Martelly and told him that the UN was "not willing to compensate any of the claimants."[67]

Not only did the UN refuse to take responsibility but it also neglected to provide support to the communities that were suffering from sickness and loss of life. Even when the disease was wiping out communities, the disease eradication work was mainly being done by local community groups and aid agencies not connected to the UN. There was widespread outrage among researchers as studies continued to build more and more evidence indicating a direct connection between the UN action (and inaction) and cholera in Haiti. Yet little was done by the UN or its local partners in response to the outbreak.

It took nearly six years and relentless pressure from researchers, epidemiologists, human rights lawyers and activists to get the UN to acknowledge its role. In 2016, the UN finally issued a vague apology that was carefully worded to avoid any legal accountability. There was no mention of the disease coming from Nepal with the peacekeepers. Ki-moon apologized to the Haitian people, acknowledging that the UN had not done enough to prevent the cholera outbreak and that it had left a blemish on the organization's reputation.[68] Critics argued that the UN's language, using terms like "moral responsibility," fell short of a full and unqualified apology that acknowledged both introducing cholera and denying responsibility for it over the years.[69] Haitians sought a more sincere acknowledgment of the UN's actions and their consequences on the country's dignity and health. Brian Concannon, the executive director of the Institute for Justice and Democracy in Haiti, a partnership of Haitian and U.S. human rights advocates, noted that the "Haitians are looking for a less qualified apology—for both introducing cholera and for the six years of denial of responsibility, which was an insult to Haitian dignity."[70]

The UN's weak response was also criticized for its lack of action and resources committed to Haiti compared with what it had done in other global health crises. This watered-down acknowledgment made global news, but things did not change on the ground. Despite the big announcements and promises, the UN and its programs did little to provide direct relief to those who were affected in Haiti.

After this non-apology, more years passed with little action. But the researchers and activists frustrated and angry about the lack of accountability and the treatment of Haitians did not give up. Finally, in May 2020, a decade after the earthquake, thirteen UN rights monitors wrote a scathing letter to the UN chief, António Guterres, for the UN's continued moral failure over the preceding decade.[71] The monitors said that not only did the UN bring a deadly disease to Haiti, it also refused to acknowledge its role for years, never fully apologized, and failed in its promises to the Haitian people. In the aftermath of acknowledging its role, the UN pledged $400 million (USD) for cholera cleanup. At the time of this writing, in 2024, it has raised only about 5 percent of the pledged funds (approximately $21 million) and spent less than 1 percent of the pledged amount ($3 million).[72]

Philip Alston, the UN monitor on extreme poverty and human rights and the lead author of the letter to the UN chief, pointed out what was clear in the minds of many: "If this happened to a white community in a country with any standing globally, the UN wouldn't have done—and wouldn't have been able to do—nothing. But this is Haiti, a country which has largely been written off."[73] Reflecting on the UN's complete disregard for the thousands of lives lost, Alston said that the UN's reprehensible conduct could only be understood by accepting that "an element of racism" played a part in it.[74]

The UN has not, to date, provided any compensation to the victims or their families. And it has shown little interest in doing so. According to a UN spokesperson, the agency is focusing on "community-based projects" instead of direct compensation.[75] Alston finds the UN's argument and line of thinking troubling. "If this happened in the United States or in Canada or in Australia and the official response was, 'We're not giving any compensation to individuals even though there was a direct link between the death of your relative and the actions of the United Nations . . . but we will build a new community home, we might set up a new health center . . .' that would be met with outrage," he said in 2022.[76]

It is important to compare the situation in Haiti—and the global response to its cholera outbreak—with how rich countries like the United States and other Western countries view "disease-carrying" immigrants. When those who are poor and dispossessed want to enter a rich country, they have been viewed as immoral, unclean, and unworthy of admission. They are seen as bringing disease to pristine lands and contaminating high culture. On the other hand, when an infectious disease comes to the poor because of the negligence and poor planning of more powerful countries and their organizations, resulting in the deaths of tens of thousands of people, no acknowledgment of the errors is made for years to come, if ever.

* * * *

HAITI IS THE most recent example of a deadly confluence of poverty, disease, and denial of care. Cholera not only devastated the country's economy and workforce but also created a permanent perception in the minds of many in the West that the country's future is permanently bleak. Poor countries are frequently denied adequate and affordable care for diseases that can be diagnosed and treated with attention and resources because powerful nations have already condemned these places to permanent misery. And then this permanent state of imported and imposed misery is used as a pretext for these nations to intervene and interfere in the poorer countries.

In 2022, as Haiti was gripped by a resurgence of cholera, the Biden administration supported a proposal to send UN peacekeepers back into the country to establish order and security there. But many Haitians had not forgotten the UN's introduction of the disease in 2010, or the organization's record of horrific sexual abuse of the local population. Mario Joseph, a Haitian lawyer who helped cholera victims, summed it up by saying, "It's really terrible. They gave us cholera, they didn't do anything to eradicate the cholera" and they are using its resurgence as a "pretext" to return.[77]

One wonders if Haiti were richer, would a similar proposal be considered seriously?

5

The Living Lab

DURING THE EARLY DAYS OF THE COVID-19 PANdemic, in early April 2020, two French physicians were talking about vaccines on television. At that time, some physicians believed that an existing tuberculosis vaccine (the Bacillus Calmette-Guérin, or BCG, vaccine) might be effective against COVID. It was, in part, driven by early data that seemed to show that people who had gotten a BCG vaccine when they were children (largely in low- and middle-income countries, since BCG is not given to children in high-income countries) were somehow not catching COVID-19. At this time of the pandemic, richer countries like Italy were facing high rates of mortality, whereas countries in Asia and Africa were doing much better. I, too, had gotten messages from family and friends in Pakistan who were pinning hopes on the vaccine they had gotten decades ago. Could BCG—a vaccine that was already available—provide a cure and stop this new and scary disease from spreading?

The initial idea was to test the vaccine in Europe, and perhaps Australia. The two French doctors, however, had something else in mind. Dr. Jean-Paul Mira, head of the intensive care unit at Cochin Hospital in Paris, casually said, "If I could be provocative, should we not do this study in Africa where there are no masks, treatment or intensive care, a little bit like it's done, by the way, for certain AIDS studies or with prostitutes?"[1] Mira's colleague, Dr. Camille

Locht, the research director of Inserm, the French National Institute of Health and Medical Research, agreed. "You are right. And
by the way, we are in the process of thinking in parallel about a study
in Africa," Locht said. The sentiment about Africa and African
bodies being a testing lab, shared by leading researchers and public
health professionals of a major European country, was met by a
fierce backlash, and the World Health Organization (WHO) called
these comments racist.[2]

For many, this statement was a painful reminder that some affluent communities continue to believe that some humans, who are
deemed less equal because of the color of their skin or their poverty, can be used as a living lab for the greater good of science.

＊ ＊ ＊ ＊

BY THE END of the nineteenth century, the mysteries around
humanity's biggest diseases, from plague to TB, were being unrav-
eled. Physicians and scientists were transforming the understanding on what causes disease. Instead of an angry god or the motion
of the stars, a living thing so small that you could not see it with a
naked eye could enter the body, undermine its immunity, stop the
organs from working, and ultimately cause death. These same agents
of disease, it was discovered, could go from one person to another
as people came into contact with each other. With this new understanding came the obvious next question: If scientific advancement can help us understand what causes infection, can it also help
us fight it? The possibility of effective therapies, rooted in the best
science of the day, was exciting for scientists and physicians, and
even for the general public.

Another group of people was also paying attention to these new
developments in science. The colonial empires of Europe had their
own reasons for wanting to get protection from and treatments for
deadly infectious diseases.[3] Western colonial powers had taken control of parts of Africa and Asia and desired to expand, or at the
very least, hold on to, these territories.[4] Infectious diseases in the

tropics threatened the colonial plunder that was essential for Western civilization to grow and flourish.

The colony of German East Africa (which comprised modern-day parts of Burundi, Rwanda, Tanzania, and Mozambique), for example, was concerned with sleeping sickness.[5] Sleeping sickness has two distinct forms of the disease and is caused by a parasite (called a *trypanosome*) that is carried and transmitted by tsetse flies. The disease is present in parts of East and South Africa (*Trypanosoma brucei rhodesiense*) and West and Central Africa (*T.b. gambiense*).[6] The symptoms of early-stage sleeping sickness include headache, swollen lymph nodes, and joint pain. As the disease progresses, it leads to confusion, sensory disturbances, and severe and uncontrolled sleep cycle disturbances (including daytime sleepiness and nighttime insomnia), hence the name of the disease.

Sleeping sickness has long been connected to the slave trade. Early observations about a neurological disease with the symptoms of sleeping sickness were made in the eighteenth and nineteenth centuries by physicians serving ships connected to the slave trade.[7] It wasn't until the first two years of the twentieth century, when the cause of the disease was identified, that the first detailed studies of the disease appeared.[8]

The mortality rate from the disease at the start of the twentieth century was significant. Colonial expansion, social restructuring, and the movement of people led to ecological changes, including forestation and deforestation, that created new reservoirs for the disease.[9] In parts of Uganda alone (which was then under British colonial rule), as many as two hundred thousand people died in the early 1900s from sleeping sickness.[10] In 1902, a church mission society noted the devastating impact of the disease: "It would be difficult to exaggerate the rapidity with which this dread scourge is spreading in Uganda and no one knows how it comes whether by mosquito as in the case of malaria in the water food or what and no one knows a cure."[11]

The high mortality rate and the likelihood of spread was of concern to colonial authorities, both in London and in Berlin. The

disease threatened the health and well-being of colonial officers and their families in the colonies as well as the ability of locals to work on farms and in the fields. With the spread of the disease, there was also concern that some regions in the colonies might become completely uninhabitable, thereby impacting agriculture and commerce.

Research in Europe on sleeping sickness was not possible as the carriers of the disease, tsetse flies, were not found anywhere in Europe and there were no reliable animal models to study the full cycle of the disease. Furthermore, the climate in which the disease manifested itself—i.e., the tropical parts of Africa—was completely different than the environment and climate in Europe.

The challenge of finding appropriate cures for the disease became a race—fueled further by scientific journals emphasizing the urgency using language that talked about colonial superiority. The British medical journal *The Lancet* noted:

> The alarming spread of sleeping sickness or human trypanosomiasis in Africa and the apparently hopeless prognosis when infection has taken place render the establishment of effective measures peculiarly urgent. . . . It is obvious that we are face to face with a real danger and that there is a need for some endeavour to stop the advance of the disease. The cause is now known and the means of combating infection are apparent it is therefore a matter for the administration of the areas in danger of infection to deal with. Neglect to carry out preventative measures must inevitably result in a loss of life among the great native populations. . . . [It is] alarming to contemplate especially when it is recalled that the disease has practically depopulated some of the districts in which it has appeared.[12]

Recognizing the potential impact of these diseases on the local workforce and its economic fallout, the colonial authorities mobilized significant funds, personnel, and other physical and material resources to tackle tropical infections.[13] Germany, being at the forefront of infectious disease research during that period, made significant investments in the effort to study sleeping sickness and find a reliable cure.[14]

The German effort was spearheaded by its most famous microbiologist and recipient of the Nobel Prize for physiology (1905), Robert Koch.[15] Koch had already made his name through his postulates of germ theory, and his discoveries concerning the microbes that cause TB (1882) and cholera (1883) made him one of the most famous scientists of his time.[16] Koch had also established himself as head of a laboratory that trained dozens of scientists who would go on to become famous in their own right. For example, Emil von Behring and his Japanese colleague, Kitasato Shibasaburo, developed treatments against diphtheria and tetanus in Koch's lab.[17] Kitasato would later be among the founders of institutes of microbiology in Japan and would shape the research on infection in his country for decades to come.[18] Koch's most famous student and mentee was Paul Ehrlich, who is widely considered the father of modern chemotherapy—the strategy using synthetic chemicals to treat diseases.[19] Ehrlich came up with the idea of a "magic bullet"—the notion that a chemical could target only the disease-causing microbe in the body, without affecting the healthy cells.[20]

Funded by the German government, Koch arrived in East Africa in May 1906 and set up his base in Bugala, part of the Ssese Islands, an archipelago on Lake Victoria in modern-day Uganda. The Ssese Islands were hit particularly hard by sleeping sickness, and between 1902 and 1908, nearly two-thirds of the inhabitants died from the disease.[21] The environment and the location, significantly different from Europe, energized Koch. Here, unlike in Germany, he had no administrative responsibilities and could exclusively focus on his work. He told his colleague, "Can you imagine a better place in the world for working? No disturbance, no visits and the mail only arrives once in a while."[22]

While the location and the mood (at least initially) was positive, to the point of being jubilant, Koch's recommended therapy for sleeping sickness was toxic. Koch had been convinced for some time that sleeping sickness could be cured by atoxyl (literally meaning *nontoxic*), a drug with a high concentration of arsenic. The drug had first been synthesized in the second half of the nineteenth century. In the beginning of the twentieth century, it had shown promise in some controlled lab studies.[23] However, atoxyl was well known to have serious side effects, even in animals.[24] Despite a lack of robust clinical data on patients and the drug's well-known toxicity in animals, Koch started his tests using atoxyl on the local African population.[25] He was convinced that atoxyl was as effective a cure for sleeping sickness as quinine was for malaria.[26]

As Koch began his work in the Bugala camp in the Lake Victoria region, word got around about a possible treatment. Patients from nearby communities, who had been suffering from sleeping sickness, started coming to Koch's treatment camp. In late 1906, the number of people seeking Koch's treatment rose to several hundred, and by early 1907, as many as 1,500 patients were in the camp. Koch started by administering atoxyl in small doses over two days, followed by a gap of a week, then giving it again for two days, and following this frequency for two months.[27] Because there was no data on what would make the right drug regimen, the protocol changed often to find the right dosage and frequency combination. Blood tests and painful injections in the back (that sometimes became infected), along with painful gland punctures, were administered to see the effect of the drug and determine the next course of action.[28]

Atoxyl—because of its toxicity against a variety of cell types—showed some early signs of success in killing the parasite.[29] However, the improvement in symptoms was only a temporary remission and not a cure. Nonetheless, Koch's apparent early success was celebrated across Europe, with *The Times* noting that the treatment was "successful in all cases."[30] This statement, by any stretch of imagination, was a gross exaggeration. And, much to Koch's dismay, the disease soon returned—often with the patient's condition worsening. Instead of recognizing that the treatment was not a cure but only a temporary respite, Koch doubled down on his treatment, believing that a higher dose was necessary for a full cure.[31] This despite previous animal studies suggesting that a high dose would result in severe side effects, including death.[32] The results of the previous animal studies did not convince Koch, however, and on some days as many as a thousand local patients and test subjects were given a high dose of atoxyl.[33] Koch's treatment was aggressive and inhumane. As one researcher working with Koch pointed out, the treatments were "not done the way clinicians used to administer arsenicals, i.e. slowly increasing doses. Instead he subcutaneously administered 0.5 each time in specified intervals over two days."[34]

The results were far from what Koch was expecting. Believing that the problem still was not a high enough dose of the drug, Koch increased it to as much as one gram of atoxyl over a seven-day period. The impact on the patients was devastating. The side effects were serious and included, among other things, an irreversible loss of sight. Koch acknowledged that "after 'some patients' had lost their eyesight irreversibly, 'the increased dose of Atoxyl was stopped immediately' and 'reduced back to 0.5 g.'"[35] Atoxyl was used along with other drugs, such as trypan red (developed by Koch's student Ehrlich)—another toxic and unsuccessful drug.[36] These treatments were so painful that the same drug could not be administered again in the same patient. Many patients—seeing the devastating consequences of the treatment—left the camp with no hope of a cure and went back to their families.[37]

Koch's campaign to treat or eradicate sleeping sickness was disastrous and unsuccessful. He noted in 1907 that "quite a few patients soon withdrew from this stronger treatment because it was too painful for them and also caused other unpleasant sensations, such as nausea, dizziness, and colicky pains in the body.

Since these complaints were only temporary, the strong treatment was continued. However, some of the patients developed a symptom which we had never encountered before, neither in the untreated patients nor in those who had not received doses larger than 0.5 g. At first, we hoped this symptom, like the others, would disappear, especially since temporary blindness had been observed several times in Europe after Atoxyl treatment. Unfortunately, there was no change in our patients, and they remained permanently blind."[38]

Koch returned from Africa in October 1907 and maintained his belief in the efficacy of atoxyl. At the same time, he argued for depopulation of the infected areas and suggested creating concentration camps. He wrote to the Imperial Board of Health in Germany stating that "one could either 'displace the entire population of the infested districts to non-infested regions. As mortality is inevitable without treatment, infected individuals would, without exception, die, the epidemic would be extinguished. . . . It is uncertain, though, whether this intervening measure could, in practice, be carried out, as it includes enormous hardships. Still, England is already endeavoring to do things along this line.' Much 'easier to pursue' and much 'more considerate' would be 'thorough examination of all inhabitants in the infested area.' Those infected would have to be 'picked out' in order to be sent to 'concentration camps.'"[39]

The term *concentration camp* was used by Koch to reference the British use of such camps in South Africa to imprison the local Boers, whom the colonial powers deemed too dangerous for mixing freely with the rest of the society.[40] It is clear that Koch was aware of such colonial practices in other parts of Africa and had no qualms about the forced separation and confinement of the local African population, going so far as to lay out where the concentration camps should be built and how many people they should hold. He also recommended to the board that in addition to creating these concentration camps, people who still got sick with sleeping sickness should be treated with atoxyl. The German public health authorities found his arguments convincing and constructed several new camps near Lake Victoria and Lake Tanganyika.[41]

In part because of his reputation and stature and in part because the Imperial Board of Health saw nothing problematic in his "pragmatic" ideas, Koch's recommendations were adopted by the board and enacted by his successor and associate, Dr. Friedrich-Karl Kleine, who took over the leadership of the German East Africa project in 1907. Kleine, a medical doctor who had studied at the University of Halle, had worked with Koch since 1900 when he joined Koch's institute in Berlin and had been part of Koch's sleeping sickness campaign since 1906.[42]

Per Koch's recommendation, concentration camps were created in the region, and as many as 1,200 patients were isolated, confined, and treated with atoxyl.[43] Kleine carried out the ideas laid out by Koch. In his mind, the concentration camps were created to take care of the "transmitters" of the disease, and atoxyl, along with other drugs, were given, in his words, "to test new drugs and do scientific research."[44] The results of Koch's treatment regimen were far from convincing. According to results reported by Kleine and his team, during 1908 and 1909, in the ten camps and six medical posts established by the German colonial authorities, only 71 of the 3,033 cases were cured, and 386 people died from the treatment.[45] The report also noted that more than a thousand patients left "for other reasons" and discontinued the treatment that was carried out at the camps.[46] Far from curing the disease, Koch's suggested therapies caused death, disability, and immense pain. Yet, little changed for years in the German colonies.

* * * *

ON THE OTHER side of the continent, Togoland was considered a "model colony," or *Musterkolonie*.[47] It had been a German empire protectorate since 1884. The region of *Musterkolonie* today comprises the country of Togo and parts of Ghana. Togoland had seen repeated outbreaks of sleeping sickness, reported as early as 1904 by German physicians in the colony.[48] As Koch experimented with his approach, his ideas about transmission and treatment reached Togoland. In this model colony, the treatment and eradication plan went further than it ever had in East Africa. Here, again, there was deep concern about the disease's impact on the economy should the local population (called *organisches Stammkapital*, or organic local capital) no longer be able to contribute their labor. When a patient with symptoms of sleeping sickness was discovered in 1908, the colonial government started an aggressive disease-eradication campaign.[49] This included testing the local population—including painful lymph punctures—and isolating and confining presumed patients. Atoxyl was given generously, and people were rounded up with the help of local police, using force if necessary. Among those in charge of the effort to combat sleeping sickness was Dr. Maximilian Zupitza.[50] Zupitza had been part of several medical missions to East and West Africa before his role in Togoland and had also been involved in suppressing the local uprisings in East Africa against German colonial rule. Zupitza knew that given the painful methods employed, patients would not come willingly to the camps or stay there. He wrote that "with the negro's lack of understanding of the village searches . . . and of other measures, with his inherent distrust of the inconvenience caused by those measures, additionally stirred up by witch doctors, passive resistance was to be expected along with attempts to 'hide the obviously sick.'"[51]

Along with coercion, Dr. Zupitza proposed creating incentives for the locals with what he called "bribes" to the families for handing over the sick. This, however, was not sufficient since there was widespread concern about the painful treatment and miserable conditions in the concentration camps. The German colonial government went further in its mission and decreed that repeated "hiding" from treatment would be met with severe punishments.[52]

In addition to testing atoxyl, Zupitza was open to using other drugs, after they had been tested on animals. The medical commission to tackle and treat sleeping sickness in Togoland started in October 1908, two years after Koch's unsuccessful attempts at using atoxyl in East Africa.[53]

The resistance from the local population was not because of the painful treatment methods alone. The history of German medical interventions also scared people off. The native population had not forgotten a prior outbreak of sleeping sickness and the subsequent forced encampment of sick patients on a mountain near Misahohé—a place that was 710 meters above sea level.[54] Every single one of those who had been sent to the camp died because of poor conditions, including inadequate and poorly constructed housing, overcrowding, lack of food, and lack of blankets and firewood in very cold weather.[55] Zupitza wrote to the governor that the high mortality in the camp was the fault of the locals, saying that the "Africans lacked understanding of the governor's intentions . . . , as well as self-sacrifice and a sense of duty towards public interests." They were also unwilling to "voluntarily put up with the interference with their personal freedom, such as treatment in the camp."[56] For good measure, Zupitza also blamed witch doctors for controlling the locals and instilling a lack of trust in the German colonial authorities.

The campaign, despite its incentives (including tax amnesty, pocket money, and tobacco for men or soap and oil for women) did not create the spirit of "self-sacrifice" that the Germans wanted to see.[57] The governor decreed that any resistance to their campaign and concealment of the disease would be met by imprisonment and forced labor for up to six weeks. Even refusal to be examined could lead to a month in prison. As a result of the new decree in 1909, disciplinary measures—including corporal punishment—could be enacted within the camp by the physician in charge and did not require authorization from the district office.[58] As a result of these drastic measures, the situation in the camps changed, but the communities outside the camps remained resistant to the colonial measures. Zupitza, recognizing that these measures were making little difference, wrote, "There is . . . always a part of the population evading the itinerant doctor, behavior that is supported by other inhabitants or even by the chiefs. . . . Those who do not feel like it are simply not at home, they are out of town. In addition, the number of doctors is insufficient. There are not enough to puncture all patients with enlarged glands let alone . . . to execute blood tests. As a result, the indigenous population understands very soon what the doctor's visit to victims of sleeping sickness is all about. As enlarged glands can easily be palpated, it is obvious that those especially who do show this symptom will do anything to avoid these examinations due to a lack of understanding."[59]

The locals tried to escape or changed their names to avoid being punished for having been in the camp and then escaped. Committed to their goal at all costs, the German physicians resorted to more and more violent methods, including chaining the feet of those who were brought to the camp. Documents from the time also show that the German doctors were far more interested in trying out various combinations of drugs to see their efficacy and doing research on their subjects than in actually caring about the disease and the suffering of the patient. German physicians working with Zupitza, such as Dr. von Raven, were clear in their goal of finding the maximum dose tolerated by the patient first— as a mission of their research—and only worrying about the efficacy of the drug and the method later, writing that "with humans the *dosis maxima bene tolerata* had to be appointed first, the most effective mode of application had to be determined in a number of experiments later."[60] To carry out these research studies, atoxyl and other drugs with high levels of arsenic were administered in higher and higher doses, and often were stopped only when the patient was considered incurable.

Haussa Naibi, a patient in one of the treatment camps, was one example. In a letter from June 1913, Dr. van der Hallen, a colleague of Zupitza's and part of the sleeping sickness commission in Togoland, wrote that as a "hopeless case he was sent back home . . . due to . . . his general condition along with the loss of his eyesight that occurred during his third Atoxyl therapy. He was no longer contagious and would not spread the plague."[61] It is likely that Naibi was just one example of many such patients who were neither curable nor of any remaining interest to the Germans.

Even after years had passed with little to show, the German physicians continued to argue for more testing, combined with successful German colonial efforts in teaching the "indigenous person to behave obediently." They proposed continued treatment with the toxic compounds and continued research with newer drugs that were being developed in Europe and suggested "extensive, time-consuming experiments" on the locals, who, in the words of Wolfgang Eckart, a prominent German medical historian, were considered the "private area" of the empire.[62]

While the extent of the outbreak in Togoland was significantly smaller than in the region near Lake Victoria, the campaign to treat or eradicate sleeping sickness there also failed spectacularly.[63] Even after the methods failed and as the local population tried to escape from the concentration camps, the proposals continued to focus on how to coerce the population, bribe potential subjects, or convince tribal chiefs. These ideas were taken seriously by German authorities in Berlin, whereas concerns about the impact of a deeply troubling, unethical, and violent campaign on population never seemed to matter very much.

More recent research on the German research expeditions in Africa has suggested a variety of motives—including pursuing personal glory, protecting the Empire's economic interests, and, above all, using some humans (those whose lives were seen as less valuable) as research subjects for finding elusive cures.[64]

The letters of German physicians from both the eastern and western edges of Africa show a deep interest in scientific progress and a strong desire for discovery of doses and treatment regimens.

Any serious concern about the well-being of the patients, or ease of their suffering, is completely absent from the correspondence.

Koch was not the only physician who had little regard for humanity when it came to studying infections. The idea that some people are naturally predisposed to infections because of their race, genetic makeup, or immoral constitution was widespread. Such people—it was believed—would make an ideal living lab, much better than a petri dish or an animal model. Because these people were viewed as less valuable members of society anyway, studying the natural evolution of disease in their bodies would greatly benefit humanity at large, with no obvious downside. The grandest experiment of this kind—with a large number of unsuspecting subjects and the full support of the state—did not happen in a European colony in Africa but in the United States.

6

We Shortened Their Lives

PETER BUXTON STARTED WORKING FOR THE U.S.
Public Health Service (PHS) in 1965.[1] PHS is the second-oldest
uniformed service in the United States, created in 1889, with its
roots dating back to the Marine Hospital Service, which was established in 1798.[2] The focus of PHS during the early days was on
quarantine and infection prevention, but over time it started to include research in other areas of disease evolution and treatment.[3]
Buxton was not a doctor or a formally trained epidemiologist but a
graduate student in history at the University of Oregon. A flier
about a job opportunity to study venereal disease took him to San
Francisco. One day, in a coffee room at his office in San Francisco,
Buxton heard someone talk about a Black patient in Alabama who
had become mentally unstable because of syphilis.[4] Syphilis was
not a new disease, or one that had the risk of overwhelming the
health system of the United States. The fact that someone had
syphilis in another part of the country, or that the disease had
reached an advanced level, was not particularly unusual. The unusual part why was when the patient was prescribed penicillin (an
antibiotic and a standard treatment for syphilis) by a doctor, someone at PHS had lost their mind. "The doctor was soon called on
the carpet by physicians for the Communicable Disease Center
(known today as the Centers for Disease Control) and reprimanded.
They said he had 'ruined their study' and 'jogged their statistics.'"[5]

This did not make sense to Buxton. How could a doctor be reprimanded for prescribing the standard treatment? Buxton was
deeply troubled and knew immediately that something was not
quite right.

Buxton's own training at PHS was about referring people for the
right treatment. Why was this particular patient being denied the
right care? And why did the Communicable Disease Center not
want this? In Buxton's mind, something was not adding up, and he
decided to look into it further. The next day, Buxton reached out
to a colleague at the CDC and was able to get several reports sent
to him.[6] The reports contained information about a study in which
patients were deliberately denied care that was available and affordable. The study crossed all boundaries of ethics. This shattered
Buxton's own notion about the organization he was part of. As he
remarked later, "I didn't want to believe it. This was the Public
Health Service. We didn't do things like that."[7] He felt compelled
to do something.

As a son of a Jewish Czech father who left Europe during the rise
of Hitler, Buxton felt a personal and an emotional connection with
the vulnerable. He started looking up what the Nazis were doing
at Dachau and Auschwitz and felt that a similar sinister mission was
at play in the United States.[8] Buxton carefully read the reports to
make sure he wasn't missing anything, then wrote and sent a report
to Dr. William Brown, head of the Venereal Disease Section of the
Public Health Service. He got no response. While the research consumed Buxton and affected him deeply, he found little sympathy
from his own colleagues. They did not want to be associated with
a whistleblower. Buxton's boss in San Francisco told him to expect
no support from his immediate supervisors. "When they come to
fire you, or do whatever they're going to do, forget my name. I've
got a wife and a couple of kids. I want to keep my job."[9]

Buxton did not want to be part of the status quo. He sent another
letter to Dr. Brown in November 1966.[10] This time, he did get a response and was asked to come to Atlanta in March 1967. Buxton was

not quite ready for what happened next. He was hoping for a discussion when he entered Dr. Brown's office; instead he was met with raw anger and verbal abuse from Brown and members of his team. The Atlanta team told him to back off from the serious work that was going on. He was told that the Black subjects in the trials were willing volunteers. Even when Buxton shared documents explicitly stating that treatment should be withheld, the team in Atlanta showed no remorse. They did show rage—but not at the injustice of the syphilis trials, only at Buxton. Despite the hostile environment, ill-treatment, and verbal abuse, Buxton did not give up.

After the death of Martin Luther King Jr. in April 1968, racial tensions in the country were at their peak. There was renewed attention paid to the historic injustice experienced by Black communities. The conversation about civil rights was no longer on the sidelines, and anger against pervasive racism in the country was palpable. Affected by what was happening in the country, Buxton wrote, once again, to the Communicable Disease Center, this time talking specifically about his moral qualms regarding the ongoing study.[11] He argued why the study was problematic to begin with since the subjects were all Black, mostly very poor, largely uneducated, and unaware of how the disease spreads. Information about the disease was withheld from them, as was effective treatment. The subjects also did not know, and were never told, the horrible effects of untreated syphilis. Information about the toll the disease would take on their bodies—and their lives—was deliberately withheld. He talked about the fact that a study of a disease that focused exclusively on a socially disadvantaged group would be unacceptable by even the most basic medical ethics standards of the time. He ended his letter by saying, "I earnestly hope that you will inform me that the study group has been, or soon will be, treated."[12]

Three months later, he received another letter from Dr. Brown, who was chairing a blue-ribbon panel "of professionals from outside the National Communicable Disease Center" to evaluate the

Tuskegee study.[13] The letter, written in a bureaucratic tone, explained that the goal of this committee was to analyze issues around "treating the remaining persons in the study group." Shockingly for Buxton, the letter concluded that "after an examination of the data and a very lengthy discussion regarding treatment, our committee of highly competent professionals did not agree nor recommend that the study group be treated."[14]

Buxton was dumbfounded. How could this study be allowed or endorsed? How could an outside panel, presumably composed of eminent physicians and public health professionals, not see what was so blatantly obvious to Buxton? And he still received very little support from his own colleagues. Buxton remained unconvinced and found the entire study morally reprehensible. He left the PHS in 1968, but his commitment to the cause did not change.

* * * *

IN 1972, AFTER a failed first attempt, Buxton was finally able to convince his friend Edith (Edie) Lederer, a journalist at the Associated Press (AP), to take a look at the syphilis study.[15] They had known each other for a few years. Buxton gave the materials he had collected to Lederer. Lederer looked at the materials and recognized that there was potentially a big story here. However, she also recognized that she was not the right person to take this assignment, but she knew someone who was. The person Edie thought could take on this assignment was Jean Heller—the only woman on the AP's special assignment team. Heller, as described by Lederer, was a terrific reporter—but the sexism of the time did not spare her, and she was described as "pixie-like" and it was noted that the AP team was made up of "ten men and one cute gal."[16]

Lederer knew that Heller was in Florida covering the 1972 Democratic National Convention that would eventually nominate Senator George McGovern as the Democratic presidential nominee to face Republican Richard Nixon. Lederer took a detour as she visited family in Florida and passed on the materials containing information about an ongoing medical study in Macon County, Alabama, to Heller in a manila envelope.[17] Heller did not get a chance to review the materials until she was on a flight back to Washington, DC. But once she read them, she was in disbelief. The detailed reports revealed that a study of the natural evolution of syphilis among Black subjects in Alabama had been going on for four decades. The government funded project tried to keep the patients from available treatment—all in the name of studying the disease in a natural environment. It was impossible for Heller to imagine that the study, which seemed so deeply flawed and un-ethical, had been going on for forty years and that it was backed by federal funds. It was also clear to her that this was not a top-secret study or a clandestine mission. Rather, plenty of people knew about it, had analyzed the data, and supported continuing the study year after year. No one among those who knew had dared, or cared, to stop it. Sitting next to Heller was the head of the investigation team at AP, Ray Stephens. She showed him the dossier. Stephens knew right away that this was serious. He told Heller to focus ex-clusively on the report once they were back in DC: "When we get back to Washington, I want you to drop everything else you're doing and focus on this."[18]

* * * *

OVER THE NEXT few weeks, Heller gathered relevant material from public libraries, medical publications, and other publicly avail-able reports. She learned that of the six hundred Black men who were enrolled, many had died and others had gotten seriously ill, as the government tried to keep them from treatment. The infor-mation given to the subjects was also incomplete; including hiding facts about the toll the untreated disease takes on the body. Others were misled and assumed that they were being treated when, in fact, they were given useless and impotent drugs. With hard evi-dence from academic journals, Heller went back to PHS. PHS was no longer able to deny or deflect. The organization finally had to own up to the ill-designed, racist, flawed, and deeply unethical study that had gone on for four decades.

Jean Heller's story appeared first in the *Washington Star* on July 25, 1972, and in the *New York Times* the next day.[19] It shocked the nation and the world.

* * * *

GERM THEORY WAS not the only major development in biology in the second half of the nineteenth century. Another tectonic movement in the field of biology came through the development and discussion around the theory of evolution. Pioneered by Charles Darwin, among others, the theory addressed competition between species, survival, and natural selection.[20] The publication of Darwin's *On the Origin of Species* in 1859 turned the world of evolution, genetic traits, and natural selection upside down.[21] Scholars and philosophers like Herbert Spencer and Sir Francis Galton expounded on the ideas of evolution beyond variations seen in birds and trees and came up with theories to explain human behavior and the evolution of societies.[22] This gave birth to the ideas that collectively came to be known as *social Darwinism* to explain the presence of the strong and the weak in society in the light of natural selection.[23] Ideas of racial superiority and hierarchy inevitably became an extension of these ideas, as did ideas of how some races were more prone to deadly diseases than others. Eugenics was a direct result of these ideas, pioneered in large part by Darwin's cousin, Francis Galton, who in 1883 defined eugenics as

> the science of improving stock, which is by no means confined to questions of judicious mating, but which, especially in the case of man, takes cognisance of all influences that tend in however remote a degree to give to the more suitable races or strains of blood a better chance of prevailing speedily over the less suitable than they otherwise would have had.[24]

In 1901 he delivered a lecture saying that

> the possibility of improving the race of a nation depends on the power of increasing the productivity of the best stock. This is far more important than that of repressing the productivity of the worst.... In seeking for the improvement of the race we aim at what is apparently possible to accomplish.... To no nation is a high human breed more necessary than to our own, for we plant our stock all over the world and lay the foundation of the dispositions and capacities of future millions of the human race.[25]

The lecture was later published in several magazines for public dissemination. These ideas of eugenics were embraced by several American physicians—some of whom were involved in creating and supporting the Tuskegee study.[26]

Against the backdrop of these ideas of inherent genetic superiority and fitness as a driver of evolution, the prevailing racism of the early 1900s saw Black people as an inferior species and tried to justify this through a variety of arguments. The idea that a Black person's body was inferior and hence prone to infection was widely accepted. Dr. W.T. English wrote in 1903 in an article titled "The Negro Problem from the Physician's Point of View" that "a careful inspection reveals the body of the negro a mass of minor defects and imperfections from the crown of the head to the soles of the feet."[27] Seven years before, in 1896, Dr. D.K. Shute had written in the *American Anthropologist* that "cranial structures, wide nasal apertures, receding chins, projecting jaws, all typed the Negro as the lowest species in the Darwinian hierarchy."[28]

The idea that Black bodies were inferior in structure was seamlessly combined with other ideas about moral values among Blacks. It was widely viewed that Black minds were inferior and simultaneously that they were plagued by immoral ideas and values. The combination of these two created, in the minds of many, a perfect breeding ground for diseases, particularly those associated with sexual promiscuity and immorality.[29]

Syphilis—a bacterial disease long associated with sexual promiscuity—was the most obvious candidate to inflict those who were genetically weak and morally compromised. While the perceived link between syphilis and immorality was held for centuries, the connection of the disease with races viewed as genetically and morally inferior only strengthened as the ideas related to social Darwinism gained traction. As early as 1906, syphilis was associated with a lack of virtue among Blacks. In the *American Journal of Dermatology and Genito-Urinary Diseases*, Daniel Quillian published a paper titled ""Racial Peculiarities: A Cause of the Prevalence of Syphilis in Negroes." Quillian argued that syphilis in Black people was a result of their inherent immorality: "Virtue in the negro race is like angels' visits—few and far between. In a practice of sixteen years I have never examined a virgin negro over fourteen years of age."[30]

Ideas such as the ones proposed by Quillian were backed by data collected over the years that showed a high prevalence of syphilis among the Black population. While the incidence was attributed to immorality and inferior bodies, the perceived consequence of the disease—poor cognitive ability, low intellect, and high crime—also fit the racial stereotypes perfectly. In 1906, Dr. Thomas W. Murrell wrote, "So the scourge sweeps among them. Those that are treated are only half cured, and the effort to assimilate a complex civilization [is] driving their diseased minds until the results are criminal records. Perhaps here, in conjunction with tuberculosis, will be the end of the negro problem. Disease will accomplish what man cannot do."[31]

Syphilis was able to capture the imagination of the public not only because of its particularly devastating effects but also because of its major mode of transmission through sexual intercourse, which was easy to blame on people who lacked virtue and existed with questionable morality.

* * * *

BEYOND THE MORALITY argument and the prevailing racist assumptions, several other factors also contributed to the start of the Tuskegee syphilis study in Alabama in 1932. First, there was a great quest to study the disease in a "natural" environment.[32] These ideas were fairly common among European and American physicians, who believed that diseases should be studied in subjects who represented a true natural experiment—one that was unaffected by treatment or technological advances. It was important that therapies should be withheld lest the pathogen adapt and make it impossible for a new therapy to be developed. It was believed that understanding how a disease evolves on its own—how it spreads and affects an individual without any intervention—would give scientists a holistic understanding of the disease, one that was not perturbed by therapies and thereby could provide them with the real Achilles heel for potent therapies.

The observation of disease in a natural environment was applied to a study of syphilis carried out at a hospital in Oslo from 1890 to 1910 on nearly two thousand patients who were denied existing therapies for their condition.[33] The lead researcher, Dr. Caesar Boeck, chief of the Venereal Clinic in Oslo, believed that mercury-based ointments and treatments, which were the only available treatments for syphilis at the time, were useless and that there was no point in giving them.[34] Boeck believed that it was better to study the disease without any treatment and see how it develops and affects the patient. In other words, his experiment was a study in the natural progression (or natural history) of disease over time and an analysis of whether the natural defense mechanisms of the body provide some kind of immunity. Researchers in the U.S. South referred to the ideas of the Oslo study several times as they developed their own program to study syphilis.[35] There was a notable difference, however. When a new drug, Salvarsan, became available and Boeck was convinced that it was a possible cure (though later studies would show that the therapy was not particularly effective), he ended his study.[36]

The notion of connecting the development of a disease, the natural environment, and the withholding of a possible cure was not limited to clinics with quarantine-like situations (as was the case in Oslo). There were other dimensions of this quest for finding cures as well, including studying a disease and giving varying levels of experimental treatment and seeing how people responded, without any real regard for their suffering. Koch's work in Africa, as we saw in the previous chapter, was part of this continuum. Researchers engaged in these kinds of studies were not particularly interested in the physical, emotional, and psychological toll on the community. Their central focus was research and their commitment was to the idea of finding a cure—with little concern for wasted bodies. Because convincing people to enroll, and to stay enrolled, was often difficult, especially as time passed, bribing them with various incentives and misleading them about the goals of the program were not viewed as problematic. The researchers were, in their own minds, pursuing the greater goal of finding a cure for a deadly disease. The cost of that mission was paid by people whose lives did not matter.

While historians believe that the twenty-year-old Oslo study had an influence on the development of the Tuskegee project, there are important differences to note.[37] The mercury-based treatments available to Dr. Boeck at the beginning of his study in the late nineteenth century were not effective therapies.[38] However, by the time the Tuskegee study was underway, the research and therapeutic landscape had changed significantly. First, the syphilis-causing bacterium *Treponema pallidum* had been identified in 1905 by two German researchers, Fritz Schaudinn and Erich Hoffmann, at the Charité (one of Europe's largest university hospitals) in Berlin.[39] A year later, a new diagnostic to detect syphilis, later called the Wassermann test, was developed by a team led by German bacteriologist August von Wassermann.[40] There were also some new treatment options available that had shown promise in animal studies, such as arsenic-based medicines that had benefited from recent developments in pharmacology, chemistry, and infectious diseases. Chief among them was the compound 606, synthesized in Paul Ehrlich's lab in 1907.[41] It was given the number as it was the six hundred and sixth compound developed for testing. The compound demonstrated antibiotic properties and was a significant improvement over mercury-based treatments.[42] It was marketed as Salvarsan in 1910 in Europe and the United States by the German company Hoechst AG.[43] Unfortunately, in addition to the painful injection process used to deliver the drug, Salvarsan had serious side effects, including rashes and liver damage. One report indicated the risk of the drug to "life and limb."[44] Regardless, it was a substantial improvement over mercury-based treatments, and when Dr. Boeck was made aware of the effects of Salvarsan, he discontinued his own two-decades-long study. He believed that there was no justified reason to deny his patients a treatment that, in his mind, was an effective cure.[45]

The idea that available treatment could be deliberately withheld was also in contradiction with existing clinical research protocols at the time. Dr. J.E. Moore, one of the leading experts in the country in venereal diseases at the time, noted in a 1933 textbook that "though it imposes a slight though measurable risk of its own, treatment markedly diminishes the risk from syphilis. In latent syphilis, ... the probability of progression, relapse, or death is reduced from a probable 25–30 percent without treatment to about 5 percent with it; and the gravity of the relapse if it occurs, is markedly diminished."[46] Demonstrating that there was somehow an exception to the rules when it came to the Black community, the same Dr. Moore, when consulted by the team organizing the Tuskegee study, was in full support of withholding treatment.[47]

The mission of the study in Tuskegee was to study the development of the disease among a rural Black community and see how untreated syphilis develops. The new project, which eventually came to be known as the Tuskegee syphilis study because of its location, had relied on the results of a previous research project that had been conducted three years before to study the progression of untreated syphilis. This project was a partnership between a Chicago-based private foundation, named after an American philanthropist Julius Rosenwald, and the U.S. Public Health Service.[48] Six counties, including Albemarle County, Virginia; Pitt County, North Carolina; Macon County, Alabama; Bolivar County, Mississippi; Tipton County, Tennessee; and Glynn County, Georgia, were selected for this research project.[49] Among these counties, Macon County had the highest percentage of men with syphilis, at approximately 40 percent.[50] The Rosenwald study suggested the possibilities of mass treatment for those who were ill and suffering among the rural Black population.[51] There was never any suggestion to simply observe the progression of disease while withholding treatment.

The specific idea for the new Tuskegee study, which was envisioned from the beginning as a "study in nature" (that is, to see passively how something happens in nature, rather than a real clinical trial with the mission of finding a cure and treatment), is often associated with Dr. Taliaferro Clark, who was one of the authors of the Rosenwald study and served as a director of the venereal disease division of PHS.[52] More recently, though, there has been some discussion that his role is probably exaggerated and that the real culprits were men at the top of the PHS bureaucracy.[53] Clark, however, made no secret of his strong opinions about the relationship between race and infectious diseases. He believed that racial factors were the cause of another one of America's public health nightmares—tuberculosis—and argued in a conference of the National Tuberculosis Association that an "inherent racial difference" made Black people more likely to contract tuberculosis.[54] Regarding the syphilis study, he wrote, "The thought came to me that the Alabama community offered an unparalleled opportunity for the study of the effects of untreated syphilis."[55] This was echoed by then surgeon general H.S. Cumming, who wrote to Dr. Eugene Dibble, a Black physician who was the head of the John Andrew Hospital at the Tuskegee Institute, "the recent syphilis control demonstration carried out in Macon County, with the financial assistance of the Julius Rosenwald Fund, revealed the presence of an unusually high rate in this county and, what is more remarkable, the fact that 99 per cent of this group was entirely without previous treatment. This combination, together with the expected cooperation of your hospital, offers an unparalleled opportunity for carrying on this piece of scientific research which probably cannot be duplicated anywhere else in the world."[56]

Surgeon General Cumming, like Clark, had strong ideas about eugenics and participated in the national eugenics movement in the United States during the first half of the twentieth century.[57] Regarding the fundamental idea of Tuskegee, Cumming noted, "It is expected the results of this study may have a marked bearing on the treatment, or conversely the non-necessity of treatment, of cases of latent syphilis."[58] Describing the situation in Macon County, Clark wrote that "this state of affairs is due to the paucity of doctors, rather low intelligence of the Negro population in this section, depressed economic conditions, and the very common promiscuous sex relations of this population group which not only contribute to the spread of syphilis but also contribute to the prevailing indifference with regard to treatment."[59]

At this time, Clark was also corresponding with Dr. Moore, who, while arguing for treating syphilis in his textbook, endorsed the idea of studying untreated syphilis. He wrote to Clark: "I think that such a study as you have contemplated would be of immense value. It will be necessary of course in the consideration of the results to evaluate the special factors introduced by a selection of the material from negro males. Syphilis in the negro is in many respects almost a different disease from syphilis in the white."[60]

Clark and Cumming were supported by another colleague with similar views on a racial basis for disease susceptibility:

Dr. Raymond A. Vonderlehr. A strong believer in the ideas of the eugenics movement, Vonderlehr was the on-site director, and he led the study team on the ground.[61] He also argued for conducting a study similar to Tuskegee among Native Americans to see how untreated syphilis developed in that community.[62] Despite his views (or perhaps because of them), he continued to rise through the ranks of the U.S. public health system and eventually became the head of the CDC in 1947.

Once the concept of the study was approved, Vonderlehr, along with Eunice Rivers, a Black nurse who had graduated from the Tuskegee Institute, canvassed Macon County for subjects who would be ideal for the study.[63] They were looking for men who were in the late stages of syphilis, could not pass the disease to their sexual partners, and were willing to be tested using the Wassermann test developed nearly a quarter century before. Unsurprisingly, few agreed. Locals were suspicious that the study had nothing to do with the treatment of syphilis but was actually a ploy to recruit for the military.[64]

Apart from finding participants, cost was a serious issue for the researchers because the study had not budgeted anything for treatment. People expected to be treated and not just tested for syphilis and then enrolled to see how the disease developed. Clark wrote to Vonderlehr, saying, "It never once occurred to me that we would be called upon to treat a large part of the county as return for the privilege of making this study. . . . I am anxious to keep the expenditures for treatment down to the lowest possible point because it is the one item of expenditure in connection with the study most difficult to defend despite our knowledge of the need therefor."[65] Vonderlehr replied,

> It is desirable and essential if the study is to be a success to maintain the interest of each of the cases examined by me through to the time when the spinal puncture can be completed. Expenditure of several hundred dollars for drugs for

these men would be well worth while if their interest and cooperation would be maintained in so doing. . . . It is my desire to
keep the main purpose of the work from the negroes in the
county and continue their interest in treatment. That is what
the vast majority wants and the examination seems relatively
unimportant to them in comparison. It would probably cause
the entire experiment to collapse if the clinics were stopped before the work is completed.[66]

To incentivize enrollment, PHS staff told the local population
that if they were ill, they would be provided treatment (which was
never the intention).[67] To keep people enrolled, Vonderlehr offered
the subjects a mercury treatment, which was well known to be
ineffective.

As the study moved forward, questions arose about the development of the disease in the body and the signs of neurosyphilis (affecting the central nervous system). At that time, there was a debate
on whether the disease affected Black people and white people differently.[68] It was assumed that Black people were going to develop
cardiovascular syphilis—which affects the great blood-carrying vessels (an argument that Vonderlehr made repeatedly)—while white
people were going to develop neurosyphilis.[69] This idea was rooted
in a belief that Black people's nervous system was unaffected by
syphilis because they had primitive brains. It was argued that Black
people had "not progressed very far from the primitive habits of
their antecedents in the rude huts of a mid-African village" and that
"temperamental and nervous defects have their influence in lower-
ing the powers of resistance and in determining the development
of tabes and the primary degenerative changes in the nervous system."[70] This idea, reflected in an essay in 1913 by Dr. E.M. Hummel,
a neurologist in Louisiana, went further to say that the disease
among white people manifested in the brain because it was the
white population "who feel the brunt of care and responsibility
greatly, and who depress themselves with the tedium of their work

and with apprehensive misgivings as to the possibility of failure."[71] The scientific advisers of the Tuskegee study believed that this research was going to settle the debate once and for all.

However, a painful procedure called a spinal tap was required for researchers to study the disease in the brain.[72] The subjects—understandably—were wary of these procedures. An elaborate scheme was then hatched by Dr. Murray Smith, head of the Macon County Health Department, whereby he sent a letter to the men who were part of the study reminding them that they had had a thorough examination already:

> Some time ago you were given a thorough examination and since that time we hope you have gotten a great deal of treatment for bad blood. You will now be given your last chance to get a second examination. This examination is a very special one and after it is finished you will be given a special treatment if it is believed you are in a condition to stand it. . . . REMEMBER THIS IS YOUR LAST CHANCE FOR SPECIAL FREE TREATMENT. BE SURE TO MEET THE NURSE.[73]

The results from the neurosyphilis study, however, were not particularly convincing. The data was messy, and not all the samples could be analyzed because they had been poorly stored.[74] The results also did not support the prevailing notion that Black communities did not want treatment.

* * * *

BY EARLY 1933, the original study was about to end and thank-you notes had been sent to the subjects, but Vonderlehr wanted to continue.[75] He wanted to see how this disease would develop in the bodies of the subjects for the next five to ten years.[76] He also wanted to conduct autopsies on the bodies of those who had died of the disease, the gold standard means of really understanding the damage to tissues and organs.[77] For Vonderlehr, the goal was to study the disease and do research, not treat those who were ill. This idea was supported by the local leadership of PHS.[78] In his communication with Vonderlehr, the regional director of Venereal Diseases at PHS, Dr. Oliver Wenger, wrote, "As I see it, we have no further interest in these patients until they die."[79]

Vonderlehr wanted to give the subjects treatments that were largely useless—like aspirins and tonics—so that they would keep coming back thinking that they were being treated.[80] Wenger was fully on board with the autopsy idea.[81] The study needed men who would not quit midway and would continue until they died. At the same time, Wenger knew that if the men realized that this project would lead to their deaths and that their bodies would then be subjected to an autopsy, they would quit.[82] A decline in the number of the subjects would undermine the whole project. To make sure this never happened, Wenger warned Vonderlehr that the men must not know that they would be autopsied: "If the colored population become aware that accepting free hospital care means a postmortem, every darkey will leave Macon County."[83] A month later, Wenger wrote again, saying, "The only way we are going to get postmortems is to have the demise take place in Dibble's hospital and when these colored folks are told that Doctor Dibble is now a Government doctor too they have more confidence."[84] Wenger wanted to exploit Dibble's trust among the local population to ensure they continued to participate in the study.

By October 1933, the new study was ready to go. A group of approximately two hundred non-syphilitic men were also selected to serve as a control group. As the new multiyear study began, the recruited subjects were never told the intent of the study or that they would never be given any treatment. Aspirin, aromatic elixir red (a red-colored solvent with no pharmaceutical properties), and other noncurative treatments were made available in sufficient quantities to give the semblance of treatment.[85] Vonderlehr, for his part, was particularly focused on ensuring that everyone who died was autopsied. He chided local doctors if they failed to do an autopsy. But families of the deceased were not in favor of autopsies of their loved ones. The PHS staff realized that resistance from the families could undermine the entire study. The matter escalated up the bureaucratic ladder. Recognizing the potential impact of resistance to autopsies on the study's outcome, Surgeon General Hugh Cumming wrote to the Rosenwald fund for support for a "burial fund," which would be used as an incentive to the tune of fifty dollars for families that agreed to an autopsy.[86] The idea for a burial fund came from the family of a deceased patient in the study.[87] The Rosenwald fund refused the request. PHS approached another foundation, the Milbank Memorial Fund, that agreed to support the project in part.[88] The fund was duly established, and families who were otherwise too poor to afford the cost of burial and desperate for a dignified funeral often agreed to accept the burial payment (a maximum of $50 to cover the cost of a casket and grave) in exchange for their agreement of the autopsies. As Eunice Rivers, the nurse who worked on the project, recalled later, "Free medicine, burial assistance or insurance . . . , free hot meals on the days of the examination, transportation to and from the hospital, and the opportunity to stop in town on the return trip to shop or visit with their friends all helped."[89]

The first research paper based on the Tuskegee study was presented in 1936 with Vonderlehr, Wenger, and Clark among the authors.[90] Although it clearly showed that syphilis, if untreated, had devastating effects on the patient, the paper did not discuss whether the patients should be provided treatment. Researchers were too consumed with the study and its results and not with the implications it may have on the bodies and lives of the subjects.[91] It was assumed as a fact that the Black participants were not to receive any treatment since no money had been set aside for treatment in the study. Throughout the study no one questioned the deception about the aspirin treatment or the misleading information. Other troubling results were also summarily dismissed. The study clearly showed that neurosyphilis was seen in a sizable number of patients (approximately 26 percent).[92] Since this challenged the prevailing race-based notions on the disease's progression (that is, that neuro-syphilis developed largely in white patients, whereas Black patients developed cardiovascular syphilis), this observation was also not taken seriously and instead was explained through a variety of con-founding and racial factors, including the presence of malaria, which was believed to affect the nervous system of Black people.[93] Overall, the study and its results were well received, and the re-searchers felt that there was no reason to stop the ongoing project.

This first publication was followed by dozens of other papers that appeared over the course of the next forty years. The Tuskegee study was not a secret, and multiple research articles showed how syphilis, if untreated, caused severe damage to the tissues and the organs. At the same time, as antibiotic treatments became widely available in 1940s, it was clear that effective treatment could make a substantial improvement in the lives of those who had syphilis.[94] Yet, the mis-sion of the study—to understand the disease in its natural form—continued uninterrupted for decades after the availability of antibiotics that were both effective and affordable.

There were, along with way, new situations that could have ham-pered the goals of the study. PHS handled these situations swiftly to ensure that nothing affected the study's mission and goals. For example, some men from the Tuskegee study were recruited by the U.S. Army during World War II. The army's policy was to start re-cruits on treatments for any ailments, including syphilis. When PHS found out that some patients from the Tuskegee study would receive treatment for syphilis, they intervened immediately.[95] They wrote to the draft board with the names of 256 people they wanted excluded from any treatment.[96] Since there were enough other men to recruit, the draft board gladly complied.

The Tuskegee study continued to deny available (and affordable) treatment to its enrolled subjects. The grand mission of research continued, even when there was no longer any doubt about the im-pact it was having. In 1950, Wenger concluded in a seminar in Hot

Springs, "We now know, where we could only surmise before, that we have contributed to their ailments and shortened their lives."[97]

Little changed in the following years. The study came up for discussion during a 1965 meeting at the CDC.[98] Race was mentioned only briefly. Despite strong evidence of the efficacy of antibiotics—that were now widely available and used for syphilis patients, not just in the United States but around the world—it was suggested that the disease in the Tuskegee subjects was so advanced that no therapy would help them. And if there was no chance of recovery, then there was no reason not to continue studying what the disease did to the body. It was also suggested that because of the abject poverty in rural Alabama, the study was actually providing them with better health care than they would receive otherwise.[99] In 1969, Dr. J. Lawton Smith, a leading proponent of the study, remarked in an ad hoc committee on the Tuskegee study at the CDC, "You will never have another study like this; take advantage of it."[100] He went further to say that "twenty years from now, when these patients are gone, we can show their pictures."[101] In this meeting, only one doctor, Dr. Gene Stollerman, argued that the patients should be treated. His objection was dismissed by the rest of the group.[102]

Though at times there were doubts about the efficacy of the study or what had been learned, there was still strong support from within the government. Dr. James Lucas, assistant chief of PHS's Venereal Disease Branch, wrote in a memo in 1970 that the study was essential and vital but also that "nothing learned will prevent, find, or cure a single case of infectious syphilis or bring us closer to our basic mission of controlling venereal disease in the United States." Regardless, in the same memo, he concluded that "the study should continue along its present lines."[103]

* * * *

WHEN JEAN HELLER'S story about the Tuskegee study appeared in newspapers in July 1972, things were continuing along the same lines as they had been over the last four decades. Autopsies on

Black bodies, ravaged by untreated syphilis, were still being performed in Macon County, Alabama. Deaths, both directly caused by
syphilis and from complications related to syphilis, were still occurring. That number of deaths is widely debated—ranging from
twenty-eight to over a hundred.[104] Heller's story sent shock waves
across the country. Yet there were doctors, even at the moment, who
put the blame on the Black subjects for not seeking treatment that
had become available. Vanderbilt University's Rudolph Kampmeier, who had served as president of the American College of Physicians from 1967 to 1968, called the outcry by journalists a tempest in
a teapot.[105] He argued forcefully that "since these men did not elect to
obtain the treatment available to them, the development of aortic disease lay at the subject's door and not in the Study's protocol."[106]
Soon after the story broke out, the U.S. Department of Health, Education, and Welfare (HEW) announced a formal review. The outcome of the review in October 1972 was the termination of the study
and the immediate treatment of the subjects. Congressional hearings, led by Senator Edward Kennedy, followed in 1973.[107]

   It took a quarter century before the U.S. federal government issued a formal apology, which was a result of the concerted effort
of many historians, journalists, public health workers and human rights advocates to correct the injustice that had went on
for four decades. On May 16, 1997, President Clinton formally
apologized for the wrong that had been committed.[108] In the audience were family members of the subjects of the study as well as
five surviving patients of the original study (out of the eight who
were alive at the time).[109] In his formal apology, President Clinton
stated that he was "sorry that your federal government orchestrated a study so clearly racist."[110] Regarding those who ran, supported, and funded the study, Clinton was clear that "they forgot
their pledge to heal and repair."[111] Unfortunately, they were not
the only group of doctors and administrators whose oath did not
stop them from inflicting harm on racial minorities who were
viewed as legitimate subjects of infection research.

7

You Know, We Couldn't Do Such an Experiment in This Country

THOMAS PARRAN JOINED THE PUBLIC HEALTH
Service in 1917, just as the United States was entering World
War I.[1] Parran worked on a rural sanitation program in Alabama
and other parts of the South. In 1926, he became head of the Venereal Disease Division (the same institution that was intimately
involved in the Tuskegee study).[2] Parran's reputation in understanding and responding to infectious diseases, particularly in rural communities, got the attention of a prominent and ambitious
governor: Franklin D. Roosevelt. Roosevelt requested Parran to
come to New York and serve as the state's health commissioner in
1930 (while still maintaining his PHS commission).[3] Soon, a New
York state commission led by Parran provided recommendations
to strengthen local health departments at the county level in the
face of severe economic anxiety caused by the Great Depression.[4]
Roosevelt wanted Parran to organize the various units of the
state's health department so that they could function better. Parran's experience in doing so served him well in the years to come.

When Roosevelt went to the White House, he tapped Parran to
coordinate federal health services. Parran was part of the committee that drafted the Social Security Act of 1935—and in particular the public health services of the act.[5] Parran continued to rise
through the ranks of government administration and in 1936 became the sixth surgeon general of the United States.[6]

Parran—because of his experience in working on infectious diseases in rural communities—had become an expert on syphilis.[7] He also recognized the stigma associated with the disease. He spoke about the disease wherever he went, to the extent that CBS Radio refused to let him broadcast because the words *syphilis* and *gonorrhea* were deemed inappropriate for live radio.[8] His book *Shadow on the Land*, published in 1937 after he had been sworn in as the surgeon general, was very well received and is still considered an important text about syphilis in the United States in the first quarter of the twentieth century.[9] Yet despite all his knowledge, awareness campaigns, and advocating for better care, Parran never asked for the Tuskegee study to be discontinued or for the patients in it to receive adequate and appropriate treatment.[10] In fact, he was an early champion of the study and thought that Macon County was an ideal location for carrying it out.[11] Instead of using his stature and understanding of the disease and its impact on people suffering from it, Parran repeatedly deferred to the regional director of Venereal Diseases at the PHS, Dr. Oliver Wenger, when it came to treatment for Black people in the study and threw his full weight and support behind Wenger's political understanding and "practical psychology" (a term Parran used to describe Wenger's views).[12] This practical psychology included ideas on how to "treat the old syphilitic with 'rheumatism', give him the painless mercury rubs. He will feel better and will bring in the whole family for the treatment they need. Don't forget, they listen to their granddaddies."[13]

There is still some debate about Parran's direct role in the Tuskegee study and how much he actually knew about its formative years (after all, he was the surgeon general from 1936 to 1948 and the study started in 1932). Recent archival research has suggested that he not only was aware but also was the intellectual godfather of the study. Philadelphia-based author and journalist Allen Hornblum argues that "if it wasn't for Parran, there never would have been a Tuskegee Syphilis Study."[14] Still, there are some who defend him or argue that he was not directly involved or perhaps was unaware, or suggest perhaps this was a misstep.[15] The defenders point to his long-term commitment to eradicating sexually transmitted infections, his deep knowledge of syphilis, and his book on the topic. While the extent of his engagement and support of the Tuskegee study may be murky, there is no debate about his role and leadership in another, even more egregious study undertaken on his watch in Guatemala.

* * * *

IN THE MIDDLE of World War II, the U.S. military was concerned with the mounting toll of syphilis and gonorrhea among its soldiers. The cost—both in actual dollars and in the loss of the men who were no longer able to serve at the front lines—was quite high. One report from 1943, for example, suggested that approximately 350,000 new infections of gonorrhea was causing the loss equivalent of putting out of action for a full year the entire strength of two full armored divisions or ten aircraft carriers.[16] The government wanted to do something to stop this loss, and among the first ideas was prophylaxis—preventing infection in the first place.

The prophylactic treatment idea was not new, and like vaccination or malaria pills to prevent disease, it was both appealing and cost effective. The National Research Council's Subcommittee on Venereal Disease agreed that a study to develop a prophylactic treatment was needed and gave it the go-ahead.[17] The doctor who led this effort was John Mahoney, a physician and a veteran of World War I who had a strong interest in venereal diseases.[18] He joined PHS, rose through the ranks, and was ultimately appointed the director of the Venereal Disease Research Laboratory of the U.S. Marine Hospital on Staten Island in 1929.[19] Dr. Mahoney was joined by a young Dr. John Charles Cutler, who was just twenty-eight years old when he joined PHS in 1942.[20] There was, however, a problem. Testing the efficacy of the prophylactic treatment meant that there should be people who are given the treatment and then deliberately given the disease. Mahoney, Cutler, and other researchers at PHS involved in the syphilis prophylactic project started looking at various options to find the right group of people as subjects for the study. Psychiatric wards were initially considered as an option but were then rejected because the researchers felt that the patients (subjects) could not fully consent to the treatment. After internal debate and discussions among the researchers, a decision was made to start the study in prisons. A federal prison at Terre Haute, Indiana, was selected as a test site.[21] The idea for the prophylaxis study was twofold. First, to see if the patients could actually catch gonorrhea when exposed directly to the pathogen, and second, to see if a prophylactic treatment would help another group of patients who had been given the treatment first and then been exposed to the disease. If successful, the study would provide the U.S. government with the clinical information and necessary tools to prevent sexually transmitted infections, particularly among its military.

To carry out the first part, in 1943–44, the researchers deposited a high concentration of *Neisseria gonorrhoeae*, the bacterium that causes gonorrhea, into the penises of 241 prisoners.[22] The results of the study, which went on until July 1944, were disappointing as far as the research team was concerned: the prisoners did not develop gonorrhea, and the Mahoney-Cutler plan was a failure.[23]

The researchers felt that the reason for the failure of the study was its inability to simulate the real scenarios—that is, the act of sex—and believed that the bacteria must be transmitted by intercourse, not by inoculation. This experiment was no longer possible in Indiana, since prostitution was illegal there.[24] But then Cutler found the perfect place to carry out the study: Guatemala. In 1945, a Guatemalan physician, Dr. Juan Funes, the chief of the Venereal Control Division of the Guatemalan public health system, was working in the Venereal Disease Laboratory on a visiting fellowship.[25] He told researchers of the gonorrhea prophylaxis project not only that prostitution was legal in his country but also that prostitutes could visit prisons.

It seemed like an ideal location. Beyond the legal cover that Guatemala provided (along with personal contacts for Cutler in the public health leadership), the country had recently gained its independence and wanted good relations with and support from the United States.[26] A grant proposal was written to continue the study with a focus on sexually transmitted infections including gonorrhea and syphilis, and the National Research Council (predecessor of the National Institutes of Health) approved funding in March 1946 for a project titled "The Guatemalan Study Dealing with the Experimental Transmission of Syphilis to Human Volunteers and Improved Methods of Prophylaxis." The total funding awarded for the project was $146,000—which would be well over $2 million by today's standards.[27] The committee that approved the funding included researchers and physicians from the nation's leading institutions, including Harvard University, Johns Hopkins University, and the University of Pennsylvania.[28]

Cutler and his team arrived in Guatemala in August 1946 and established a field site.[29] The supplies needed to continue the lab work were supported by the U.S. military transport. By early 1947, Cutler had made lots of friends in powerful circles. He started enacting his plan for intentional exposure (sexual intercourse) in the country's largest prison, Penitenciaría Central. Sex workers were intentionally exposed to gonorrhea by inserting gonorrhea pus into their vaginas.[30] As a result, all of the sex workers in the study got infected. The infected sex workers were then made to have sex with uninfected men. In some cases, the sex workers were required to have sex with many men in a row.[31] In one instance, one woman had sex with eight men in a period of a little over an hour.[32] Despite this, the disease transmission rates remained low.[33] Overall, the results were quite disappointing, with less than 10 percent of the men getting infected.[34] Cutler and his team soon expanded the research subjects to include soldiers, inmates in the only psychiatric hospital in the country (Asilo de Alienados), and even children in an orphanage (who were included to study congenital syphilis). These subjects were never told that they were part of an experimental study.[35]

For those who developed the disease, it was not clear whether the treatment they were given was adequate or that the disease was cured. The case of Maria Luisa, a commercial sex worker, is particularly telling. Maria was paid $25 in March 1947 for her role in the study (i.e., having sexual contact with seven men). In the following months, Maria was inoculated eleven different times with gonorrhea. She was given different strains of the disease and was made to have sexual contact 105 times during this period. A later report noted that "there is no evidence that Maria Luisa received any treatment for her acute gonorrhea during the experiments."[36]

With overall results still not what Cutler was looking for, he resorted to even more extreme methods. He started injecting infected pus directly into the urethra of the subjects. Berta, a female patient at the psychiatric hospital, was injected with gonorrhea (gathered from an infected male) in her rectum and eyes. Cutler and his team also infected her with syphilis. Berta died three days later.[37]

The extreme measures adopted by Cutler and his team led to an increase in infections among his subjects. To see how the infection was developing (or not developing), painful lumbar punctures (removal of the spinal fluid) were performed.[38] For recordkeeping, serial photographs were also taken of the subjects.[39] To get a deeper understanding of how infection spread, Cutler's team tried a variety of modes of infecting individuals, including infecting the eyes of the men who were enrolled in the study. In addition, for some patients, reinfection studies were performed, including "surgical removal of penile chancres."[40]

As both gonorrhea and syphilis were of interest to the U.S. team, extreme measures were also employed to infect patients with syphilis. In one particular case, Cutler made women in the study drink syphilitic solutions.[41] He also tried to develop a human model of neurosyphilis by injecting syphilis infection directly into the spinal fluid of the subject. According to the records, 1,308 people participated in the study.[42] A report by the Presidential Commission for the Study of Bioethical Issues studying the Guatemala studies noted that "not only is there no record of consent to participation in the experiments, there are also several examples of active deceit on the part of the researchers."[43]

Beyond the deeply unethical practice that took away the agency and autonomy of the persons involved and egregiously exploited several vulnerable groups, all in the name of preserving resources for the U.S. military, the research also did not provide any valuable scientific information. The inhumane measures to create infection were far from realistic scenarios of how disease spreads in reality, and the so-called realistic scenarios failed to create disease among the subjects.

Cutler and Mahoney both knew that their work was unethical, and they did not want the word to get out. An article in the *New York Times* in April 1947 by journalist Waldemar Kaempffert said that any plan that would "shoot living syphilis germs into human bodies" would be unethical.[44] When Cutler saw the article, he got concerned. Referring to the *Times* article, Cutler wrote to Mahoney on May 17, 1947:

> It is becoming just as clear to us as it appears to be to you that it would not be advisable to have too many people concerned with this work in order to keep down talk and premature writing. I hope that it will be possible to keep the work strictly in your hands without necessity for outside advisors or workers other than those who fit into your program and who can be trusted not to talk. We are just a little bit concerned about the possibility of having anything said about our program that would adversely affect its continuation.[45]

A month later, on June 22, 1947, he again wrote to Mahoney:

> As you know it is imperative that the least possible be known and said about this project, for a few words to the wrong person here or even at home might wreck it or parts of it. We have found out that there has been more talk here than we like with knowledge of the work turning up in queer places.[46]

Dr. R.C. Arnold, who was the director of syphilis research at the Venereal Disease Research Laboratory, was involved from the beginning of the project, and had visited Guatemala on April 14, 1948, wrote to Cutler, "I am a bit, in fact more than a bit, leery of the experiment with the insane people. They cannot give consent, do not know what is going on, and if some goody organization got wind of the work they would raise a lot of smoke."[47]

* * * *

WHILE CUTLER WAS the person on the ground, and Mahoney the overall head of the Guatemala program, the effort was fully supported by Surgeon General Thomas Parran. Parran was supportive of the study in federal prisons when it was first started and subsequently approved the grant in April 1946 to start the project in Guatemala. He was well aware of the goals and approaches used in the studies. Mahoney wrote to Cutler in October 1946 that "Doctor Parran and probably Doctor Moore might drop in for a visit after the first of the year."[48] Dr. Joseph Moore was the head of the review committee at NIH that had approved the grant, among the leading experts on venereal disease in the country, and a faculty member at Johns Hopkins University School of Medicine. It is the same Dr. Moore who in 1932 had written that "syphilis in the Negro is in many respects almost a different disease from syphilis in the white."[49] In December 1946, Mahoney wrote to the team in Guatemala that "the Surgeon General has become keenly interested in the Guatemala project."[50]

Archives of letters and statements from Parran (and his close colleagues) clearly demonstrate that not only did he support the Guatemala project but he also knew that the entire enterprise was deeply unethical. In a letter to Cutler, a PHS official wrote, "I saw [surgeon general] Doctor Parran . . . and he wanted to know if I had had a chance to visit your project. Since the answer was yes, he asked me to tell him about it and I did so to the best of my ability. He was familiar with all the arrangements and wanted to be brought up to date on what progress had been made. As you well know, he is very much interested in the project and a merry twinkle came into his eye when he said, "You know, we couldn't do such an experiment in this country."[51]

When Parran stepped down in 1948, Mahoney knew it was time to wrap up the work and clean up the tracks. He wrote to Cutler that they had "lost a very good friend" (referring to Parran).[52] He then instructed Cutler to "get our ducks in line."[53] Mahoney also said, "We feel that the Guatemala project should be brought to the innocuous stage as rapidly as possible."[54]

The project folded soon afterward, but the reports were never published and were largely forgotten until a Wellesley College professor, Dr. Susan Reverby, saw something unusual while she was researching Parran's role in the Tuskegee trials in 2003.[55] Reverby is a distinguished historian who has written extensively on the Tuskegee study.[56] During her research of the Thomas Parran archives at the University of Pittsburgh, a colleague informed her of the papers of John Cutler that were also housed at the university. Cutler was also involved with the Tuskegee study in the 1960s.[57] The box containing Cutler's documents actually contained nothing on Tuskegee (which is what Reverby was looking for) but instead had extensive documents on a Guatemala study that Reverby knew almost nothing about.[58] The documents revealed both the extent of the study and the deeply unethical practices that went on with the full support of the government, including that of Surgeon General Thomas Parran.

As a scholar who had worked on the history of the Tuskegee study, Reverby could see both the similarities and the differences in the two studies. Both studies shared the fundamental assumption that race and infection were interconnected. In other words, members of certain racial groups developed different kinds (or severity) of infectious diseases based on their race. But unlike the Tuskegee study, which was about seeing how latent syphilis develops if left untreated, the project in Guatemala focused on *giving* people the disease. Reverby had worked for decades trying to present a clear picture of the Tuskegee study, dispelling the myth that Black sharecroppers were deliberately infected (they were not). "I've spent 20 years of my life saying to people nobody was [intentionally] infected in Tuskegee and I open up this box sitting in your archives—and here is this inoculation study and it's Cutler," she said in an interview in 2011 (and recounted to me when I spoke to her in March 2024).[59] Reverby sent her findings to the former head of the CDC, David Sencer, whom she had gotten to know during her research.[60] Shocked by what he saw, Sencer told his CDC colleagues about it. The CDC sent its own team to Pittsburgh to review the archives and make their own judgment.[61] They came to the same conclusion Reverby had, which triggered a chain reaction that went from the CDC to the NIH and all the way up to President Obama's desk. In October 2010, the United States formally issued an apology through a joint statement from Secretary of State Hillary Clinton and Health and Human Services secretary Kathleen Sebelius: "Although these events occurred more than 64 years ago, we are outraged that such reprehensible research could have occurred under the guise of public health. We deeply regret that it happened, and we apologize to all the individuals who were affected by such abhorrent research practices."[62] President Obama also apologized to his Guatemalan counterpart Álvaro Colom.[63] A bioethics commission—established by executive order of the president—concluded that "the Guatemala experiments involved unconscionable basic violations of ethics, even as judged against the researchers' own recognition of the requirements of the medical ethics of the day."[64]

After the formal apology, several lawsuits were filed against the U.S. government, as well as against the pharmaceutical company Bristol-Myers Squibb, Johns Hopkins University School of Medicine, and the Rockefeller Foundation, for compensation and damages.[65] The lawsuits continued for several years before being dismissed by judges in favor of the defendants. The judges ruled that U.S. institutions were not liable for the damages caused to the Guatemalan people.[66] To date, no compensation has been made to the victims or their families.

The architects of the Guatemala program not only did not face any questions but also continued to enjoy prestige in their disciplines and the support of their peers. They were showered with coveted awards and held leadership positions. John Mahoney was given the Albert Lasker Award for clinical research in 1946 for his "pioneering the treatment of syphilis with penicillin."[67] After he retired from the Public Health Service in 1949 (the Guatemala study had been quietly wrapped up a year before), he became the health commissioner of New York City. Mahoney died in 1957.[68]

After stepping down from his role as surgeon general, Thomas Parran went into academia and became the inaugural dean of the School of Public Health at the University of Pittsburgh, where he stayed until 1958.[69] The main building of the school was named Parran Hall in 1969.[70] Things changed, however, half a century later. As Reverby uncovered more evidence of Parran's role in Guatemala, public health scholars, who had long considered Parran a hero, were faced with a dilemma. How does one square his contributions (including his work in crafting the Social Security System and destigmatizing sexually transmitted infections) with his direct knowledge and support of the syphilis and gonorrhea studies in Guatemala?[71] The report of the Presidential Commission for the Study of Bioethical Issues in September 2011 left no doubt in the minds of public health scholars of Parran's involvement in the despicable acts committed in the name of research and scientific discovery. While several public health, history, and political science scholars tried to paint the Tuskegee and Guatemala studies as missteps in an otherwise extraordinary career of a remarkable public servant, others expressed disgust for Parran's role in them.[72] Students, faculty, and staff at the University of Pittsburgh felt strongly that the fundamental mission of public health—taking care of all people with the highest principles of ethics and humanity—was at odds with Parran's legacy and that having his name on the building that houses the School of Public Health was antithetical to the values of the discipline. The movement gained momentum, found support from the school's dean, Donald Burke, and was reviewed by a university committee. The review, which included analysis of historical documents and community discussions, eventually led the university's chancellor, Patrick Gallagher, to acknowledge Parran's involvement in studies that "conducted human trials on vulnerable populations without their informed consent—actions which are fundamentally at odds with our own core values as a leading research university."[73] On June 29, 2018, the trustees of the University of Pittsburgh voted to remove Thomas Parran's name from the building that houses the public health program.[74]

John Cutler—the main architect of the Guatemala studies—took part in additional projects conducted in the name of science, discovery, and disease and remained committed to his idea of injecting patients with infection, seeing how the infection develops, and then analyzing the efficacy of available treatments. One such project (conducted with another colleague, Sidney Olansky) was an infamous study at Sing Sing prison in New York in 1955 in which prison volunteer inmates were deliberately given syphilis and then treated four months later to study reinfection and response to treatment.[75]

Cutler's role in the Tuskegee study is also worth mentioning. He became assistant surgeon general in 1958 and got involved with the

Tuskegee study in the 1960s.[76] Given his interest in syphilis and the potential therapeutic power of antibiotics (particularly penicillin) in treating syphilis, he knew very well what the Tuskegee study was and how it was being carried out. The argument against treating participants in the early phase of the study was that treatment for syphilis was expensive and hence outside the study's limited budget. But by the time Cutler became involved, penicillin was widely available and affordable in the United States, and yet he never made any efforts to offer antibiotics to the patients in Alabama.[77]

Cutler continued to rise through the ranks of the U.S. public health bureaucracy. After his stint as assistant surgeon general, he had a distinguished career at the University of Pittsburgh, where he also served as an acting dean of the School of Public Health.[78]

Even after the Tuskegee study was discontinued in 1972, Cutler continued to defend the goals of the study and showed no remorse for his involvement in it. In the 1990s, Cutler told a news reporter that "Tuskegee was undertaken for the highest ethical reasons."[79] In a PBS *Nova* documentary that aired in 1993, Cutler said, "It was important that they were supposedly untreated, and it would be undesirable to go ahead and use large amounts of penicillin to treat the disease, because you'd interfere with the study."[80] Cutler emphasized that the Tuskegee subjects were in fact saving others, saying that "some will die. It is in the interest of the total society. These men in Tuskegee helped us learn how to treat syphilis among blacks. They were serving their race."[81] According to him, the Black men enrolled in the Tuskegee study were serving as "controls for the entire race."[82]

Cutler was never asked questions about the Guatemala study. He died in 2003 before his role became public in 2010. His obituaries praised him, calling him a pioneer in the prevention of sexually transmitted diseases. Quotes by colleagues included statements such as Cutler "thought every person should have access to these services, regardless of income."[83] The *Pittsburgh Post-Gazette*, the main newspaper of the city where Cutler had lived and worked for the last thirty-five years of his life, while noting all Cutler did for global health did not even mention the word *Tuskegee* in its obituary even once.[84]

8

Bacteria as a Bomb

BY THE END OF THE 1930S, A COVERT LAB IN NORTH-eastern China was the center of a top-secret Japanese defense program. Located in the city of Harbin, the capital of Heilongjian province, the lab became the central research facility to develop a new kind of weapon.[1] It was well supported in material and human resources and housed thousands of researchers.[2] The lab consisted of fifty buildings surrounded by a wall and a dry moat as well as high-voltage wires. The lab also had a railway siding, an animal house, an airfield, and a block (called *Ro*) that was used for human experiments.[3] The lab's main goal was to create biological and chemical weapons for the Japanese Imperial Army. These weapons were duly tested on the local Chinese population that was under Japanese occupation at the time.

* * * *

THE LAB IN Harbin was nicknamed Unit 731 and was led by General Shirō Ishii, a microbiologist and senior officer in the Japanese Imperial Army. Shirō was born in Japan in 1892 and graduated from Kyoto Imperial University in 1920, after which he joined the Army Medical Corps.[4] He traveled through Europe and the United States with the goal of learning about the West's latest weapons technology and the use of bacteriological weapons in

World War I. He was appointed as a professor of immunology at the Tokyo Army Medical School and given the rank of major.[5]

Armed with the latest ideas about European weapons, Shirō convinced the Japanese military leadership to invest in a biological weapons program.[6] In 1932, he was appointed to a testing and production facility located in Manchuria, a Chinese province Japan had invaded the prior year.[7] Under Shirō's leadership, the biological weapons program became more formal and structured and toward the end of the decade had greatly expanded its mission.[8] The program not only manufactured biological weapons but also tested them on the Chinese villagers under the Japanese occupation.[9] As had been the case in Africa and Asia where colonizers (Europeans) exploited the colonized for resources, labor, and expansionist interests, here, too, a colonized community (the Chinese) was on the receiving end of a program created to support the political and military goals of the colonizer (Japan).

* * * *

OFFICIALLY NAMED THE Epidemic Prevention and Water Purification Department of the Kwantung Army, Unit 731 was a busy place under Shirō, who was well connected within academic and political circles in Japan.[10] Throughout the late 1930s and during World War II, Shirō continued to move up the ranks and eventually became surgeon general. Aided by strong connections in the military and the imperial court, Shirō and his supporters convinced hundreds of doctors and other military personnel from various medical schools to work on this cutting-edge scheme to create biological weapons and test their efficacy on live humans.[11]

Unit 731 was involved in torturing not only captured men and women but also babies who were born as a result of the systematic rape of Chinese women in the region.[12] It is now known that Unit 731 was not the only facility to develop and test biological weapons, but it was certainly among the most prominent. Like military research facilities elsewhere, the unit was supported by similar smaller laboratories in cities across China.[13]

The clandestine lab's first focus was humanity's old scourge, the bubonic plague.[14] By this time in the 1930s, it had been well established that the plague spread through the bite of infected fleas. Building on the research on plague of the prior decades, Unit 731 started breeding plague-infested fleas in the lab.[15] These fleas were then spread in several Chinese cities as well as ports and coastal areas by air.[16] Low-flying airplanes dropped paper bags filled with the plague-infested fleas in Ningbo and Quzhou in Zhejiang province.[17] Plague-infested rats were also let loose in several Chinese cities.[18] This was accompanied by deliberate denial of care by the Japanese authorities to the infected patients, who were desperate to seek treatment for a disease that rained down on them.[19] The result was catastrophic, with thousands of fatalities in villages and cities.[20]

These plague-infested-fleas-in-bags were not the only trials conducted on unsuspecting Chinese civilians. To test the efficacy of waterborne agents as biological weapons, marshes, wells, and reservoirs in rural China were infected with anthrax, cholera, and typhoid agents.[21] Unsurprisingly, cholera killed scores of locals, who were unprepared for the outbreaks.[22]

Shirō, based on his record in China, planned an attack on Californian cities with biological weapons as well. According to the plan, bombs containing millions of bubonic plague–infested fleas and other biological agents were to be deployed using Kamikaze pilots in an operation code-named Operation PX, or Operation Cherry Blossom at Night.[23] Many years later, in 1977, Captain Eno Yoshio, who was involved with the planning of the operation, recalled,

The plan was not put into actual operation, but I felt that just the fact that it was formulated would caused [sic] international misunderstanding. I never even leaked anything to the staff of the war history archives at the Japanese Defense Agency, and I don't feel comfortable talking about it even now. But at the time, Japan was losing badly, and any means to win would have been all right.[24]

The plan never went ahead because of opposition from the chief of army general staff, General Yoshijirō Umezu, who had concerns about bacteriological warfare getting out of hand.[25]

By the end of World War II, as many as two hundred thousand Chinese civilians had been killed as a result of biological warfare testing and use, and the epidemics of cholera, plague, and anthrax that followed the attacks.[26] These numbers are comparable to the deaths caused by atomic bombs in Hiroshima and Nagasaki.[27] Despite the enormity of the crimes and the scale of casualties, information about Japan's war crimes using biological weapons was actively suppressed by the Allied Forces in the postwar tribunals.[28] During the Tokyo tribunals, Shirō and his team received full immunity.[29] The United States negotiated the immunity deal in these trials in exchange for information from the biological weapons programs.[30] The U.S. leadership wanted to learn more about the technical details of the program and use that research for their own military purposes.[31] Historians believe that General Douglas MacArthur, in charge of the Tokyo tribunals, was well aware of the immunity deal and suspect that he may even have negotiated the terms.[32] He made it clear when he wrote to Washington, DC, that "additional data, possibly some statements from Ishii probably can be obtained by informing Japanese involved that information will be retained in intelligence channels and will not be employed as 'War Crimes' evidence."[33]

* * * *

DESPITE HIS CENTRAL role in crafting and leading the biological weapons program and testing biological agents against Chinese civilians, Shirō continued to live peacefully in Japan after the war and died in 1959 from throat cancer.[34] His other colleagues involved in biological weapons research and development went on to have prosperous and successful careers in Japan that ranged from the governorship of Tokyo to leadership of the Japan Medical Association and the Japanese Olympic Committee.[35]

* * * *

UNIT 731 WAS most likely the first instance where biological weapons were actively used against civilians, and it was certainly one of the largest state-sponsored projects of its time. But the idea of deploying germs and toxins on the battlefield had been around for some time before that. As the germ theory of disease became well established, researchers and military strategists started to imagine how they could use it for military purposes. They were interested in whether conventional weapons could carry germs as their payload. Since weapons programs are often clandestine, a detailed history can only be pieced together from archives and later interviews of those who were involved in these weapons developing programs.

Historians believe that the first established program was probably in France in the interwar years, in particular the 1920s.[36] It was led by French chemist Auguste Trillat, who focused on weapons that could use airborne pathogens, which are stable in the atmosphere and could be dropped from the planes.[37] The Trillat program ran well into the late 1930s in France and was only closed down under German occupation during World War II.[38] For most of the 1920s and 1930s, the United States and Britain were not particularly interested in biological weapons—not because of any serious moral qualms but because they felt that these weapons were unreliable and less effective compared to chemical weapons.[39] The Allied stance, however, changed as war with Germany loomed. Canadian pharmacologist Frederick Banting, who had received the Nobel Prize in 1923 for the discovery of insulin, dismissed the idea that airborne pathogens made for weapons were too fragile and unreliable. In 1939, he argued for using all means necessary to disseminate germs, including postal mail if necessary. He also had no issues with attacking civilian targets and factories. Banting argued,

> In the past, war was confined for the most part to men in uniform, but with increased mechanization of armies and the introduction of air forces, there is an increased dependence on the home country, and eight to ten people working at home are now required to keep one man in the fighting line. This state of affairs alters the complexion of war. It really amounts to one nation fighting another nation. This being so, it is just as effective to kill or disable ten unarmed workers at home as to put a soldier out of action, and if this can be done with less risk, then it would be advantageous to employ any mode of warfare to accomplish this.[40]

Banting was not the only one with this idea of all-out war. He had plenty of supporters in the United States and Britain who believed the same.[41] The enemy had to be destroyed, and biological weapons offered new possibilities to accomplish this goal. If that required disabling the workforce and terrorizing the population, then so be it.

During World War II, the United States started its own biological weapons program and provided resources to allies (in particular to the United Kingdom) in their own pursuit of biological weapons. Aware of the developments in biological weapons among other countries, the U.S. Secretary of War, Henry Stimson, in 1942 requested that the U.S. National Academy of Sciences provide its scientific input on the matter.[42] In a letter to the president of the academy, Stimson wrote,

> Because of the dangers that might confront this country from potential enemies employing what may be broadly described as bio-

logical warfare, it seems advisable that investigations be initiated to survey the present situation and the future possibilities. I am therefore asking if you will undertake the appointment of an appropriate committee to survey all phases of this matter. Your organization already has before it a request from the Surgeon General for the appointment of a committee by the Division of Medical Sciences of the National Research council to examine one phase of the matter.[43]

* * * *

BY 1943, THE United States had officially started its biological weapons program in Camp Detrick (later Fort Detrick) in Frederick, Maryland.[44] Through this program, a large production facility was built that was supported by field testing sites across the United States (including in Pine Bluff, Arkansas, and Dugway Proving Ground, Utah).[45] Researchers, physicians, and microbiologists brought their cutting-edge knowledge of disease and pathogens to the U.S. war effort, describing in research papers, briefs, and memorandums the behavior of various promising pathogens under particular environmental conditions and their suitability for maximum impact on a target population.[46] One report that came out during this period is particularly noteworthy.

In 1942, two Columbia University researchers, Theodor Rosebury and Elvin Kabat, wrote a report on the use of biological weapons.[47] Like Trillat and Shirō before them, Rosebury and Kabat were experimental lab scientists, aware of the research findings made by their peers around the world and well versed in the fundamentals of germ biology. But Rosebury and Kabat were not just academic researchers. They were also directly involved in the U.S. war effort. Rosebury served as the division chief of the biological weapons program at Camp Detrick, and Kabat, the younger of the two, was involved in the program as a consultant for the U.S. Army.[48] Overall, their report demonstrated a more sophisticated understanding of biological warfare agents than what Trillat had achieved a decade and a half earlier and what the

Japanese were experimenting with in Unit 731. Their fifty-page report describes why some specific pathogens could actually be a very effective weapon of war and achieve objectives that conventional weapons could not. They argued that in addition to biological agents being capable of diffusing over large areas of land, they also had the capability to "psychologically frighten" the civilian population in the enemy territory.[49]

* * * *

THE ROSEBURY-KABAT REPORT also sought to systematically and clearly differentiate between biological and chemical weapons.[50] This was an important issue to focus on at the time, since most weapons programs until that point often lumped these two kinds of weapons together. The authors noted several distinctive features of biological weapons. These included the fact that biological agents, unlike chemical weapons, have an incubation period. Not all pathogens make a person sick immediately. This meant that unlike chemical weapons, which make an impact relatively quickly, biological weapons may take days (or more) to affect the target population. Incubation periods also vary with different pathogens, and hence offer a wide variety of options, depending greatly on the mission.[51]

The second major difference was the contagious nature of biological agents. Once deployed, they can pass from one person to the other, either through direct contact or through other means, including air and water. Unlike chemical weapons that do not have a life of their own, biological weapons can proliferate and affect communities beyond the original target. While Rosebury and Kabat did not mention this in their report, the implication of these agents becoming endemic in a community and affecting generations is clear.

Third, Rosebury and Kabat pointed out that unlike chemical weapons, biological weapons are characterized by infectivity, which is a measure of the frequency of inducing symptoms.[52] This infectivity was not simply the measure of how potent the weapon was or the concentration of the agent; rather, it depended on impacted individuals and the likelihood that they would get sick. Some people in the target population could have natural immunity and may not be seriously affected, while others may get really sick very quickly. Finally, Rosebury and Kabat noted that perhaps the greatest advantage of biological weapons over chemical weapons was that the former did not need to be manufactured from basic elemental constituents.[53] The agents existed in nature already, and under the right conditions, which could be created in labs and manufacturing facilities, they could grow and proliferate on their own. At the same time, the two scientists were also cognizant that many biological agents needed a mammalian host to survive and thrive and that without a host, they were unstable and, perhaps, unusable on the battlefield.

A major contribution of the Rosebury-Kabat report was a systematic ranking of pathogens in terms of their potency, their ability to withstand battle scenarios, and their longevity. The authors were clear in the mission of biological weapons for the military and wrote that these weapons were "for the disorganization of industrial areas behind the lines or of army centers and camps; for use as a part of 'scorched earth' policy, and against valuable animals, food plants and industrial crops."[54] With this in mind, they reviewed seventy potential pathogens as biological weapons agents. These agents were, by then, well-known disease-causing pathogens, and there was sufficient information about their fundamental biology (such as their life cycle, needed growth conditions, and likelihood of surviving in various climates and conditions) as well as whether the diseases that they caused could be treated.

Rosebury and Kabat analyzed the suitability of the pathogens to be used as weapons on the basis of ten characteristics.[55] These included the ease of availability or cultivation; the ease of dispersal (aerial or otherwise); the impact the agent would have on the population (in terms of what percentage of the population might get sick, or even die); the ease or difficulty in developing effective defense against the disease caused by the agent (i.e., how fast could the enemy forces or the local population develop immunity or defenses against the disease); and, perhaps most ironic of all, the long-term impact the agent might have on friendly troops who might later occupy the area.[56]

* * * *

APPLYING THESE TEN characteristics to their original list yielded thirty-three likely and potential pathogens and thirty-seven rejected pathogens.[57] Despite decades of research and new knowledge since the time of their report, the pathogens Rosebury and Kabat analyzed in the 1940s would still be listed, decades later, as the most lethal agents for biological warfare.[58]

At the top of the Rosebury-Kabat list was anthrax.[59] Anthrax had been a common disease, particularly in animal farms in Europe. Robert Koch, a pioneering microbiologist of the late nineteenth and early twentieth centuries, came up with his ideas on germ theory through working with cattle that had died of anthrax. Anthrax inhalation deaths had been reported in the early twentieth century in textile industries that processed goat hair, goat skin, and wool. While incidences continued to decrease over time with better industrial hygiene practices, the death rate for those who inhaled anthrax remained extremely high (85 percent or more).[60] Anthrax was attractive to Rosebury and Kabat for a variety of reasons: It can be spread over great distances and its spores are hardy and can handle changes in air pressure as well as high and low temperatures. Rosebury and Kabat wrote that it was "surpassed by few microorganisms in infectivity for animals, and by none in host range."[61]

* * * *

PLAGUE WAS ALSO rated highly in the Rosebury-Kabat report.[62] The bacteria that cause plague could be dispersed as an aerosol, and it showed outstanding stability in lab conditions that simulated the harsh battlefield environment. Rosebury and Kabat wrote, "There is no reason to doubt that virulent plague bacilli could be disseminated by the airborne route, and that under conditions which can be rather clearly defined, a devastating epidemic could result."[63] Rosebury and Kabat were most enthusiastic about the same two diseases, namely anthrax and plague, that had been identified by Shirō's unit 731 as the most promising for killing, maiming, and terrorizing large populations. Like the Japanese in China, Rosebury and Kabat also discussed deploying various infectious agents through mosquitos, fleas, ticks, and other insects.[64]

Beyond anthrax and plague, a few other pathogens were also listed as effective options. These included tularemia—or rabbit fever that can lead to sepsis and death.[65] Also mentioned was brucellosis, a bacterial disease that can cause fevers, back pains, and damage to the central nervous system.[66] The symptoms and resulting illness can last for years.

The Rosebury-Kabat report is not particularly long, at approximately fifty pages. It is also not written as a scientific paper or a policy brief. Instead, it reads like a manual on how to choose the best biological weapon agent for a particular purpose. There is, however, a clear tension throughout the report between good public health practices, which both Rosebury and Kabat were aware of because of their clinical training and practice, and the desire to exploit weaknesses in the public health system for the purposes of inflicting damage, pain, and destruction among vulnerable enemy populations. This idea is sometimes referred to as "public health in reverse."[67] The goal of this *mission in reverse* is to hit the maximum number of people with disease and illness, rather than protecting them from harm and providing them with health care against disease. Talking about this tension, Rosebury and Kabat wrote,

For the student of bacterial warfare the emphasis shifts fundamentally. He is concerned with the weak links only in order to strengthen them, or to discard the whole chain if they cannot be strengthened. He is much more interested in the inception of mass infections than he is in the details of their perpetuation, except, of course, that for the purpose of defense against bacterial warfare, or for control of mass infections once they have begun, he must fall back on the knowledge of the whole epidemiologic chain.[68]

At the end of the war, in 1945, Rosebury went back to medical research and wrote a series of influential pieces for both the research community and the general public, including a widely acclaimed book.[69] His postwar stance and opinions were similar to that of many who had worked on clandestine, highly destructive weapons-making projects during the war. He now feared a world where weapons like the ones he worked on would become widely available and cause immense pain and destruction. Soon after his departure from Camp Detrick, Rosebury became a strong advocate against biological weapons. His 1949 book *Peace or Pestilence?* provides a clear and candid account of how biological weapons are developed and their potential risk against unsuspecting and vulnerable populations. His own experience added both credibility to this account and a recognition of what was possible. The book became popular and was reviewed positively in the academic and popular press.[70]

* * * *

IN MAY 1942, several years before the publication of Rosebury's book, President Roosevelt had approved the imposition of serious restrictions on public discussion and disclosure of a national program "to create an organization within the Federal Security Agency to conduct the U.S. Biological Warfare Program."[71] Following the war, the United States faced new enemies. Soon, the Cold War was in full swing and the fear of a possible Soviet attack dominated policymaking. In 1946, General Eisenhower, then the head of the U.S. Army, banned any disclosures regarding the biological weapons program and imposed an injunction against any official mention of the term *biological warfare*.[72] In 1949, Secretary of Defense

James Forrestal said on record that the U.S. program was meant only to protect the U.S. population against the Soviet threat. He did not mention the offensive goals of the program.[73]

While Rosebury became an advocate for caution and restraint, his co-author, Elvin Kabat, came under an increasingly common attack in postwar U.S. politics: he was accused of being a Communist.[74] Interestingly, it was the Rosebury-Kabat report, which became publicly available right after the war, that was used as a basis for *Time* magazine to suggest that Kabat was an enemy sympathizer and that he was publishing classified information. Soon after this accusation, the FBI opened an investigation on Kabat and started reading his mail. This was, however, only the beginning, with worse yet to come. A former colleague of Kabat's, Professor James Sumner, told the FBI he suspected that Kabat was a Communist sympathizer. At the height of McCarthyism and the Red Scare, this accusation was enough to derail the career of anyone, regardless of their contributions to national security or their work during the war. That is exactly what happened with Kabat, who was pressured to resign from his position at the VA hospital.[75] He was also barred from traveling internationally for several years, until the restriction was finally lifted in 1955.[76] At the same time, the Public Health Service refused to renew Kabat's grants.[77] They were not concerned with the merits of his research, just with his reputation. They were uncomfortable supporting the research of anyone who might be a Communist, or a Communist sympathizer. To resolve this issue, the Public Health Service suggested that the work could continue with someone else as the lead researcher. Kabat refused and was ostracized from the research community for several years.[78]

Given the political climate and the anxiety about an all-out war with the Soviet Union, the United States continued to develop strategies for the effective development of biological weapons in classified programs for well over two decades following the end of World War II.[79] This was despite the fact that the science was clear

and unambiguous: the technology that was being developed was
not only going to harm and inflict unbearable pain on unarmed civilian populations but also could easily trigger long-term epidemics, which could become very difficult, and costly, to control.

* * * *

THE ETHICS OF causing harm to others was not a particularly
prominent concern in military circles. While there were naysayers
of biological weapons, their main concern was that these weapons
might not be as reliably effective as they were claimed to be. Resources could be better spent elsewhere, they argued, and in the
absence of more convincing results that could prove the battle
readiness of biological weapons, they called for either severe
budget reduction or a complete shutdown of the biological weapons program.[80]

The scientists, doctors, and military personnel committed to developing these weapons had two strategies to address the reserva-
tions of the pessimistic leadership within the military.[81] The first
was to improve the quality of the field tests. They had to demonstrate that the aerosols containing pathogens could be spread
over a wide area of enemy territory, including densely populated
urban targets, in varying weather conditions.[82] Strong field data
would build confidence about the reliability of the weapons and
prove that the weapons could reach their target and could be used
reliably and repeatedly in all kinds of terrain.

The second strategy involved showing that these biological weapons could actually cause the desired damage. Here, the approach
from the developers was to perform tests on human subjects to get
convincing data. Human subjects would be exposed to varying
doses of pathogen-containing aerosols, simulating various wartime
scenarios envisioned by the military. The developers intended to
minimize risk to the subjects and avoid long-term sickness or death
by administering recently developed antibiotics, either as a prophylactic or as a postexposure treatment.[83]

As part of these efforts, a number of experiments and field sim-
ulations were carried out. The developers pursued their two strategies of proving effective field coverage and human response,
separately and, in some cases, together. Since the likely adversary
was the Soviet Union, simulation exercises and field tests were carried out with that region's terrain and weather conditions in mind.
A new project, called the St. Jo Program, was launched in 1953 by
the U.S. Army Chemical Corps (which ran Camp Detrick) to
study how an aerosol attack on enemy territory could unfold.[84] The
St. Jo Program focused on simulating anthrax attacks on large Soviet urban centers. St. Louis, Minneapolis, and Winnipeg, Canada,
were chosen to model Soviet cities.[85] The plan was for the operatives to release noninfectious bacteria from generators mounted on
top of cars, while local authorities were informed that "invisible
smokescreen[s]" were being deployed to obscure the cities from
enemy radar.[86] The next phase of the program tested the dispersal
patterns of particles released from airplanes to assess the weapons'
impact on even larger areas. The Large Area Concept experiment
took place in 1957 and involved the dispersion of microorganisms
across a wide area from South Dakota to Minnesota. According to
the army, these experiments "proved the feasibility of covering large
areas of the country with [biological weapons] agents."[87] Data from
these studies included information on air dispersal patterns, potential exposure (using simulants that mimicked anthrax spores),
and the impact of weather on the dispersal and spread of the spores.
The data was then used in a mathematical model to predict "casualty production" in enemy territory.[88]

The army didn't acknowledge the St. Jo Program, and its release
of 239 germ warfare tests in open air between 1949 and 1969, until
1977.[89] When the report finally came out, they also acknowledged
that they had released microorganisms at Washington National
Airport in 1965 and in the New York subway during peak hours in
1966 to study how spores would spread and how effective this type
of attack might be in densely populated areas.[90]

The biological weapons program was also not immune from egregious episodes of racism at the time. In 1951, the army released a biological warfare agent called *Aspergillus fumigatus* at the Norfolk Naval Supply Center.[91] The pathogen was well known to cause immunodeficiency and could lead to lethal infections. This particular pathogen had also been known to tolerate high heat and could remain active and stable even at 122°F. At the naval supply center, where the pathogen was released, most of the workers were Black. This was not a coincidence but based on racist assumptions about Black bodies being different (and inferior) than white bodies when it comes to immunity or the likelihood of infection. Long-standing views about why Black people get sicker from diseases like smallpox or syphilis were, once again, at play here. A report about the test plainly stated that "since Negroes are more susceptible to coccidioides than are whites, this fungus disease was simulated by using Aspergillus fumigatus."[92]

While the St. Jo Program tested coverage, questions remained about human infectivity, dose response, and tolerance. To get reliable data in order to address these questions, the military embarked on Operation Whitecoat.[93] The idea was to expose military members with a toxin, for which there were effective antibiotics, and study how well they would tolerate exposure to the pathogen and how the disease would develop despite having access to antibiotics.[94]

Operation Whitecoat was not simply going to address skepticism within the military about biological weapons—it was also aimed at developing the military's own data on human subjects. There were already concerns within some military circles that the Soviets were launching an unethical human subjects study and were therefore going to have highly relevant data for creating more sophisticated and potent biological weapons.[95] The United States could not afford to fall behind.

* * * *

IN 1952, PHYSICIANS at Camp Detrick in Maryland came up with a plan to start tularemia exposure on human subjects. The proposal was initially met with resistance from military personnel at Camp Detrick and resulted in a sit-down strike.[96] In response, the designers of the program came up with another idea: to enlist Seventh-day Adventists (SDA), conscientious objectors who had joined the military under the condition that they would not bear arms (that is, they would serve as noncombatants) but could work as medics.[97] In 1953, with the help of SDA church leaders, the project started under the code name CD-22.[98] This time, the pathogen of choice was a bacterium named *Coxiella burnetii*.[99] This bacterium is responsible for Q fever, or Query fever, which produces flu-like symptoms. From the testing standpoint, it was an attractive choice for two reasons. First, its spores could be created in the lab with relative ease. These spores could then be inhaled by the volunteers, mimicking the real-world scenario of biological warfare. Second, the illness responded well to antibiotics. Having effective and rapid treatment options readily available was going to build confidence and avoid the risk of adverse outcomes. The pilot study started with ninety volunteers, and the results around inhalation and treatment were highly promising, showing that the disease could in fact be spread by desired means and, when needed, could be treated by appropriate therapies. A larger study could now commence.

The plan for the next stage was to work with a larger group of volunteers for a longer period of time and with a more aggressive pathogen. *Pasteurella tularensis*, which causes tularemia (rabbit fever), was chosen for this purpose.[100] This bacterium is easy to aerosolize and is highly infectious. If untreated, however, tularemia is lethal. The properties of the bacterium, and the resulting disease, were well known in infectious disease circles and had resulted in it being ranked high as a potential weapon in the Rosebury-Kabat report of the 1940s.

With the help of the Seventh-day Adventist Church, the U.S. Army trained conscientious objectors, who were medics and had volunteered for the program.[101] During the project, the subjects were observed for their response to antibiotics and their ability to perform simple daily tasks, including basic mathematics.[102]

Over the course of the twenty-year program, which came to a close in 1973 with the ending of the draft, nearly two hundred human subject tests were conducted.[103] More than two thousand volunteers, most of them SDA church members, participated in the study.[104] The effects of the disease were varied. Some volunteers took a few days to recover, while others were sick for weeks and took a long time to be completely free of the disease. The U.S. Army claimed that there were no long-term effects of exposure and that everyone recovered completely.[105] Some of the volunteers, however, disagreed and claimed that negative effects of the experiments, including back pain and heart ailments, continued for a long time.[106]

Over the years, Operation Whitecoat has been hailed as an example of humane human subjects research, an example of informed consent, and an effort well ahead of its time.[107] This view, however, remains contested. While consent forms were provided, the intent of the project was never transparent. The volunteers and church leaders understood the project to be purely defensive in nature and its main goal to build a strong defense against the country's enemies. As stated by a former volunteer, "By using these individuals as 'human guinea pigs' military medical personnel were able to demonstrate the feasibility of preparing a defense against biological warfare agents and known risk factors that existed not just in the battlefield, but also in the workplace."[108] However, there is good reason to be skeptical about the stated mission. The project was not just about developing a defensive strategy to protect soldiers and civilians. In fact, it was to develop an offensive weapon, something that was not clearly articulated to the volunteers. Many volunteers remain upset about this breach of trust.[109]

During the 1960s, the line between research to defend the country and its people and research to kill the unarmed citizens of an enemy country became fuzzy. Field testing of new weapons continued to increase, driven in part by the military's engagement in

Southeast Asia and the need for newer weapons in Vietnam. During the same time period, new developments in computing, mathematics, material sciences, and chemistry allowed for better packaging of biological agents and provided high-quality data on the longevity of biological weapons and their range of impact.

A new Department of Defense project, called Project 112, was authorized by Secretary of Defense Robert McNamara in 1962 to test biological and chemical weapons, including in land and sea testing sites.[110] The program, which ended in 1973, was multinational and involved collaboration among the departments of defense of the United States, Canada, and Britain.[111] Some of the Project 112 tests were indeed meant to examine defensive capabilities, but the majority were designed to simulate the bombing of enemies and included testing biological warfare in environments similar to what U.S. forces were seeing in Vietnam. One series of experiments, called the Yellow Leaf trial, focused on how well aerosolized biological (and chemical) weapons could penetrate a jungle canopy similar to that found in the tropical environment of Vietnam.[112] These tests were conducted first at the Fort Sherman military reservation in Panama and then in Hawaii.[113] There was, of course, no reason to do these tests if the mission was purely defensive. No large U.S. population centers are located in or around a dense jungle canopy.

During the two decades after World War II, the biological weapons program benefited from the U.S. military's chemical weapons program, either by having joint testing sites or by utilizing prior knowledge gained from nuclear testing undertaken in far-off islands.[114] Other tests, such as Magic Sword (1965), focused on the dispersal of infection using mosquitoes.[115] Tests of tularemia as a biological warfare agent were conducted at Fort Greely in Alaska (1963–65), where the environment and climate were similar to those of cities in the Soviet Union.[116]

* * * *

JUST WEST OF the International Date Line, and a few degrees north of the equator, is a country composed of a group of Micronesian islands, collectively known as the Marshall Islands. The Marshall Islands include over two dozen atolls, which are ring-shaped islands or coral reefs. The United States, after gaining control of these islands from Japan in 1944, conducted sixty-seven different nuclear tests there over a twelve-year period, from 1946 to 1958.[117] It was in the Marshall Islands in 1952 that the United States tested the most powerful weapon of its time, the hydrogen bomb. The testing site was the Enewetak Atoll. To carry out the test, which was code-named Mike, some of the local population was forcibly removed from the main islands.[118] The thermonuclear tests resulted in significant environmental damage to the region. The test also had a severe impact on the health of the local population.[119] As part of the research, the U.S. military relocated the removed communities back to the islands where the nuclear tests had been carried out so researchers could study the long-term impact of the bombs' aftermath on humans. The health of the local population was never a serious concern to the U.S. military. The locals were, in the words of those responsible for the tests, not quite civilized. Merril Eisenbud, an officer with the U.S. Atomic Energy Commission, made his views clear during a meeting in January 1956: "While it is true that these people do not live the way that Westerners do, civilized people, it is nonetheless also true that they are more like us than the mice."[120] Unsurprisingly, reports over the ten years after the tests were carried out showed a significant rise in cancer, miscarriages, and birth deformities.

Beyond the consequences for human health, there is also the issue of the lasting impact on the environment. Today, the structure, commonly referred to as "the Tomb" by the locals, has become vulnerable to rising sea levels.[121] The contamination of the land and the destruction of its native flora and fauna continues to trouble the local community to this day. But the asymmetric power dynamic between these islands, which are poor and in need of aid, and the United States, which is a provider of that aid, affects the outcomes of any discussions between the two countries.

* * * *

WHILE THE NUCLEAR tests in the Marshall Islands formally stopped in 1958, the U.S. military did not share with the locals any information about a series of biological weapons testing that was carried out there a decade later, in 1968. In September and October of 1968, without prior information or consent, the U.S. military performed some of its most elaborate biological weapons tests at the same location it had carried out the hydrogen bomb test: Enewetak Atoll.[122] This series of biological weapons testing was called DTC 68-50.[123] The pathogens in these tests were some of the nastiest agents that had been tested to date. The payload included Staphylococcal enterotoxin B.[124] This particular pathogen is known to cause severe toxic shock and food poisoning and is considered among the most potent biological warfare agents. The Staphylococcal enterotoxin aerosols were sprayed using McDonnell-Douglas F-4 Phantom jets. The goal of these tests was to measure the efficacy of the agent and its capacity to spread over a very large target area. To achieve this goal, the jets were fitted with a new dissemination tank called the AB45Y-4. This device was long, thin, and pointed and resembled a V-2 rocket. The jets were piloted by U.S. Air Force Vietnam War veterans. The complete records of the tests remain classified, but one unclassified paragraph describes the success of the mission:

In the summer of 1968, the Deseret Test Center conducted a series of tests known as DTC 68-50 from the USS *Granville S. Hall*, anchored off Eniwetok Atoll. This test series involved the atmospheric dissemination of "PG"—*Staphylococcal* enterotoxin Type B—a toxin that causes incapacitating food poisoning that causes flu-like symptoms that can be fatal to the very young, the elderly, and people weakened by long term illness.

Staphylococcal enterotoxin B was disseminated over a 40–50 km downwind grid, and according to the Final Report, a single weapon was calculated to have covered 2400 square km, an area equal to 926.5 square miles.[125]

The unclassified paragraph is significant for several reasons. First, it is clear that this was no defense exercise. Second, the description of the capacity and range of a single weapon is extraordinary. The area covered, 2,400 square kilometers, is about the size of metropolitan Moscow or about double the size of Los Angeles. The fact that this agent was stable and would stay potent for some time is also noteworthy. In cities with high population density, millions could become ill. So is the fact that the agent would have the greatest impact on the most vulnerable persons, including babies and the elderly, as well as people who were sick, lacked adequate access to good health care, had a weak immune system, or suffered from underlying health issues.

* * * *

GIVEN THE POTENTIAL of inflicting serious and long-term harm to the enemy troops and to citizens living in the enemy territory, the United States was not the only country to weaponize its medical and biological science research and create biological weapons. As a matter of fact, it was a latecomer to this effort. The United Kingdom, for example, was well ahead of the United States and had conducted field tests of anthrax bombs on Gruinard Island, an uninhabited island on the northwest coast of Scotland, in the early 1940s.[126] The strains of anthrax used in the tests were supplied by Professor R.L. Vollum of Oxford University—and hence were named Vollum 14578 in his honor.[127] These strains were already among the most lethal anthrax strains, and through a process of natural selection became more and more virulent as they were exposed to more hosts (that is, animals and humans).[128] The British anthrax tests, which killed nearly all the sheep that were brought to the island and tethered near the bomb's landing site, were at least a hundred times more potent than any chemical weapons of the time.[129] Small, oval-shaped Gruinard Island, where the anthrax experiments were carried out, remained contaminated with anthrax spores for nearly five decades, despite repeated attempts to clean it. One such effort included setting fire to the whole island. That attempt was a failure.[130] Despite the fire, the spores remained intact and potent.

Even at the height of World War II there were concerns about the short- and long-term impact of biological weapons. In response to these questions, Paul Fildes, a pathologist and former head of the UK Medical Research Council's bacterial chemistry unit, who was recruited to lead the secret program developing and testing biological weapons, wrote, "Is it any more moral to kill Service men or civilians with HE (High Explosives) than with BW (biological weapons)? . . . It seems clear to me that a substantial majority of the population would conclude that, if they had to put with a war again, they would prefer to face the risks of attack by bacteria than bombardments by HE."[131]

* * * *

THE UNITED STATES, the United Kingdom, and Canada were not the only countries recruiting scientists and physicians into their national programs for developing and testing biological weapons. While the U.S. program ended with a speech from President Nixon on November 25, 1969, the Soviet Union continued its own program.[132] The research to develop biological weapons in the Soviet Union started well before World War II and continued in various research units throughout the 1950s and 1960s.[133] The most elaborate effort to consolidate various programs and systematically create biological weapons was through the establishment in 1971 of a Soviet agency named All-Union Science Production Association, or Biopreparat (Biological Preparation).[134] Among the visionaries for this industrial-scale, highly secretive operation was a young star of the Soviet science establishment, Yuri Ovchinnikov.[135]

A graduate of Moscow State University, Ovchinnikov was a biochemist with an interest in genetics.[136] At forty, he became the vice president of the USSR Academy of Sciences, an unusual achievement in a country where it was rare to be in the upper echelons of any organization until one was much older.[137] Given his party credentials and strong support within the organization, he had the ear of Soviet leadership.[138] Ovchinnikov was able to convince Leonid Brezhnev, general secretary of the Communist Party, that Soviet science lagged behind the West in many critical areas, including genetics, biochemistry, and molecular biology. The failure to keep up not only had implications for the reputation of the Soviet Union but also had significant implications for its military.[139] These conversations led to the creation of Biopreparat in 1974.[140] This was significant on two levels. First, this effort was a violation of the 1972 Biological Weapons Convention that had outlawed biological weapons.[141] Second, the national program came at a time when basic scientific understanding about pathogens and their toxins, along with clinical understanding of virulence and human immune response to disease-carrying viruses and bacteria, had become highly sophisticated. Antibiotics were available and were being widely used. Improved diagnostics for infectious diseases were also becoming cheaper and more available in countries across the world.

Driven by the conviction that the Soviet Union needed to be ahead of its adversaries in biological weapons and aided by a broader understanding of disease, Biopreparat brought together the military, the Soviet Ministry of Agriculture, the Soviet Ministry of Health, and the KGB.[142] Many of Biopreparat's employees were scientists and clinical researchers who had been working in university labs.[143] The size of the program was significant, and research, development, and testing facilities were dotted all over the Soviet Union, from Moscow to Kirov to Kazan. At its peak, as many as thirty to forty thousand people worked in the program.[144] As in the United States and the United Kingdom, the biological weapons program was also closely affiliated with the chemical weapons program.

Yet despite its size and the involvement of multiple ministries, Biopreparat remained largely a secret. The West did not learn of its existence or its scale until the late 1980s, and in more detail after the collapse of the Soviet Union in 1991.[145] Since then, interviews of researchers who worked in Biopreparat have started to paint a picture of a program that was extraordinary in scale and scope.[146] The pathogens that were developed as weapons largely mirrored the efforts in the United States. Anthrax—once again—was of great interest to Soviet authorities.[147]

The USSR anthrax biological weapons program, designed to harm enemy citizens, resulted in a major accident that killed dozens of Soviet citizens. The tragedy unfolded in Sverdlovsk, a city nearly 1,500 kilometers east of Moscow, now called Yekaterinburg.[148]

During the Soviet years, Sverdlovsk had become a manufacturing hub, and industries associated with the military found a home there. As Biopreparat became operational, Sverdlovsk received its share of biological weapons production sites. In April 1979, weapons-grade anthrax aerosols were accidentally released from one of the production sites.[149] Dozens of people died and several thousand became seriously ill.[150] The United States found out about the anthrax outbreak in early 1980 and publicly raised its concern in March 1980.[151] The Soviets did not deny the outbreak but linked it to human consumption of infected meat.[152] Beyond the back-and-forth between the two global superpowers of the time, the issue did not get much traction until after the collapse of the Soviet Union, when, in 1992, U.S. scientists, along with local Russian researchers, found out the exact nature and extent of the outbreak and were able to link it directly to the covert military production site.[153] The final confirmation came from Boris Yeltsin, president of the Russian Federation, who, in May 1992, announced that the military was responsible for the anthrax epidemic.[154] Yet, no one in the military or the government was held responsible.

* * * *

FOR NEARLY FIVE decades, countries in Asia, Europe, and the Americas developed biological weapons—using fundamental discoveries in biological, physical, and health sciences to create lethal instruments of war. The same discoveries that could, and did, save millions of lives were weaponized in an out-of-control arms race. The purpose of biological weapons was—first and foremost—to inflict harm on innocent civilians. In the case of Japanese war crimes in China, hundreds of thousands became victims of these instruments. But in other parts of the world, innocent people paid a direct and indirect price as well. The exact numbers of those whose lives were affected may never be known.

9

Infection and the Border, Revisited

THE RIO GRANDE FORMS A CRESCENT AS IT FLOWS southeast from its source in the San Juan Mountains of south central Colorado, through valleys and canyons, forests and deserts, and passes through New Mexico, Texas, and the Mexican states of Chihuahua, Coahuila, Nuevo León, and Tamaulipas for nearly two thousand miles before reaching the Gulf of Mexico.

Supporting the lives and livelihoods of nearly 6 million people and home to diverse flora and fauna, the river has served as a border between Texas and Mexico since the Treaty of Guadalupe Hidalgo in 1848 that ended the Mexican-American War (1846–48) and resulted in the United States gaining control over California, Nevada, Utah, and New Mexico.[1]

In the mid-nineteenth century, river crossings from the north to the south were a ticket to freedom for those trying to escape slavery in the United States. The risk to those trying to escape west or far north out of Texas, which had joined the United States as a slave state after winning its independence from Mexico in 1836, was substantial.[2] But going farther south, to Mexico, where slavery had been outlawed in 1837, offered some hope.[3]

An informal network of informants and resources created a southbound underground railroad. This network was smaller and more informal than its northern counterpart, but it included information about abolitionists and pathways that people could use to cross into Mexico. Enslaved persons, in search of freedom, used any and all means available to them, including wagons of cotton and horses, to traverse the vast southern landscape until they reached Mexico.[4]

Felix Haywood, a former slave and a resident of San Antonio, Texas, noted in 1937 (when he was ninety-two) that "there wasn't no reason to run up north. All we had to do was to walk south, and we'd be free as soon as [we] cross[ed] the Rio Grande. In Mexico you could be free."[5] Felix further said, "Sometimes someone would come 'long and try to get us to run up North and be free. We used to laugh at that. . . . They didn't care what color you was, black, white, yellow or blue. Hundreds of slaves did go to Mexico and got on all right. We would hear about 'em and how they was goin' to be Mexicans."[6] In time, U.S. enslavers in the South recognized this avenue to freedom and brought it up with Mexican authorities, asking them to return "their property."[7] The Mexican authorities did not comply.[8]

Today, most river crossings are in the other direction, and the reception north of the border is far from welcoming. Individuals and families crossing the river into the United States are seeking freedom from gang violence, urban conflict, corruption, and crippling poverty that are in part caused by a series of coups (that were at times supported by the U.S.) that derailed democracy in the region and made the way for dictators and despots to stay in power for decades.[9] Migrants trying to reach safety are met with U.S. border agents who can permanently change their lives in an instant.[10] Border agents have tremendous power over the lives of migrants; they can detain migrants, force people to return to the violent neighborhoods they were escaping from, and they can trash or confiscate medicines if they choose to.[11] Border agents routinely separate families, making arbitrary and impulsive decisions that result in permanent separation between parents and young children.[12]

The treatment of asylum seekers and migrants at the southern U.S. border has progressively gotten worse in the last three decades.

During a debate between presidential candidates Ronald Reagan and George H.W. Bush in 1980, a question was asked about undocumented migrants coming from Mexico.[13] Both future presidents, Reagan and Bush, argued for more acceptance and inclusion. Bush called the undocumented "honorable, decent, family-loving people," and Reagan argued for open borders on both sides, saying, "They can cross and open the border both ways by understanding their problems."[14] This conversation would be unimaginable today—in either Republican or Democratic debates. Since the 1990s, several policy changes have resulted in greater incidences of violence against migrants. In 1994, a "prevention-through-deterrence" strategy was adopted by the U.S. Border Patrol, which led to an increase in the number of border agents and the active patrol of urban crossings.[15] The agency's budget increased from $326 million in 1992 to over $4.6 billion in 2019, and the number of agents has increased fivefold.[16]

Curbing immigration has become a major topic in local and national political campaigns. Phrases such as "tough on crime" and "law and order" are used in conjunction with "closing the borders." With immigration as the centerpiece of policies during the first Trump administration, the COVID-19 pandemic provided the government with a legal basis to turn people back at the southern border. Part of the law that provided the legal cover to the government in 2020 was passed in 1944. It is commonly known as Title 42.

* * * *

THE STORY OF Title 42 goes all the way back to the 1930s. The New Deal and World War II profoundly impacted the public health landscape of the United States. Federal and state administrations recognized that the existing systems of disease surveillance and health care access were dated and in need of an overhaul.[17] New developments in science and technology—from lab tests to drugs—required a system that could cope with changes in diagnosis, treatment, and management at the population scale. Consequently, there was a significant increase in the budget and a several-fold increase in the staff of the U.S. Public Health Service (PHS).[18] Despite its growth, or perhaps because of it, the system was badly in need of reorganization and integration. The public health system of the time was siloed, and the mandates of various administrative units within this system were unclear. New programs for disease control and eradication, from malaria to typhoid and from sanitation to community health, had little direction or guidance.[19] Thomas Parran, the surgeon general under Roosevelt (and whose role in Tuskegee and Guatemala was discussed in previous chapters), had spent his career in public health and was aware of the system's messiness. His team was routinely criticized for the chaos that ensued at PHS. In response, Parran, with support from the White House, assembled a team of lawyers, congressional staffers, and PHS officials that sifted through "100 years' worth of earmarked acts, appropriations measures, Presidential Executive Orders, and regulation."[20]

The result was the passage of two acts by the U.S. Congress. The first was the 1943 Public Health Service Act (78-184), signed by President Roosevelt in November 1943 and designed to "cast PHS as a tightly knit bureaucracy by career health professionals." The second was the Public Health Law (78-410), signed in July 1944 and which "codified the agency's legislative bases, creating a statute that would become an operating backbone of PHS."[21] These two acts are enacted in Title 42 of the U.S. Code. (The U.S. Code refers to the general and federal statutes of the United States.) Title 42 broadly deals with public health, social welfare, and civil rights.[22]

Title 42 is long and full of legal jargon. It has 164 chapters, and each chapter has multiple subchapters and clauses. But there is one particular clause that became the basis for the U.S. government to deny asylum rights at the border. This clause is in Section 265, Part G, Chapter 6, and subchapter IIA. It states the following:

> Whenever the Surgeon General determines that by reason of the existence of any communicable disease in a foreign country there is serious danger of the introduction of such disease into the United States, and that this danger is so increased by the introduction of persons or property from such country that a suspension of the right to introduce such persons and property is required in the interest of the public health, the Surgeon General in accordance with the regulations approved by the President, shall have the power to prohibit, in whole or in part, the introduction of persons and property from such countries or places as he shall designate in order to avert such danger, and for such period of time as he may deem necessary for such purpose.[23]

In 1966, the authority described in the clause was transferred from the surgeon general to the director of the U.S. Centers for Disease Control and Prevention (CDC) as part of the reorganization of PHS.[24] For decades, Section 265 of Title 42 remained buried deeply in the annals of U.S. code. The idea of invoking it was first considered in 2018 but it did not gain much traction.[25]

* * * *

IN MARCH 2020, during the early stage of the COVID-19 pandemic, when the idea for Title 42 was put forward by members of the Trump administration, CDC scientists and public health experts were not convinced that it would work or that it was even the right policy. They had supported the proposal for a nonessential travel ban, but putting a complete stop to all asylum applications and turning everyone away at the border, including unaccompanied children, was viewed as unnecessary.[26] The suggestion that the arrival of migrants at the border was somehow the source of new coronavirus cases in the United States was not substantiated by data from either Canada or Mexico.[27] Undeterred by epidemiological evidence or advice from senior public health leadership, the administration pushed. Vice President Pence told the CDC director, Dr. Robert Redfield, to enact Title 42. On the phone call to Redfield in March 2020, Pence was joined by his chief of staff, Marc Short, and acting secretary of U.S. Department of Homeland Security, Chad Wolf.[28] Both Short and Wolf put pressure on Redfield, despite resistance from senior CDC leadership, to use the act to shut down the borders completely. Redfield eventually complied and told his staff to "get it done."[29]

While Mark Morgan, the acting head of the Customs and Border Protection, said that "this is not about immigration. What's transpiring right now is purely about infectious disease and public health," several CDC officials disputed this claim both publicly and privately.[30] Martin Cetron, director of the CDC's division on global migration and quarantine, later told the Congress that the CDC had no role in pushing for enactment of Title 42 and that it "came from outside the CDC subject matter experts."[31]

Soon after the order to enact Title 42 was issued, Customs and Border Protection offices quickly started implementing it. The CBP's website was also quickly updated:

On March 21, 2020 the President, in accordance with Title 42 of the United States Code Section 265, determined that by reason of existence of COVID-19 in Mexico and Canada, there is a serious danger of the further introduction of COVID-19 into the United States; that prohibition on the introduction of persons or property, in whole or in part, from Mexico and Canada is required in the interest of public health. Under this order, CBP is prohibiting the entry of certain persons who potentially pose a health risk, either by virtue of being subject to previously announced travel restrictions or because they unlawfully entered the country to bypass health screening measures. To help prevent the introduction of COVID-19 into border facilities and into the United States, persons subject to the order will not be held in congregate areas for processing and instead will immediately be expelled to their country of last transit. In the event a person cannot be returned to the country of last transit, CBP works with interagency partners to secure expulsion to the person's country of origin and hold the person for the shortest time possible. This order does not apply to persons who should be excepted based on considerations of law enforcement, officer and public safety, humanitarian, or public health interests. Expulsions under Title 42 are not based on immigration status and are tracked separately from immigration enforcement actions, such as apprehension or inadmissibility, that are regularly reported by CBP.[32]

The enactment of Title 42 led to the rapid expulsion of individuals and families who had shown up at the border, without giving them a chance to apply for asylum in immigration court. There was no due process, regardless of the strength of the claim or risk to the life of the individual if they were to be sent back.[33] Over the course of the next few months, between March and October of 2020, two hundred thousand migrants and asylum seekers were sent back to Mexico.[34]

Initially designed to be in place for just a month, Title 42 was first extended for one month by Redfield and then enacted for an indefinite period in May 2020.[35] During the next three years (that included over two years of the Biden administration), migrants at the southern border were repeatedly ill-treated. A report by Physicians for Human Rights noted that "in one terrifying incident, a mother described Border Patrol agents intentionally capsizing and destroying an inflatable raft that was holding a group of migrants, including small children."[36] A mother who crossed the border near Reynosa, Mexico, recounted,

> All the mothers were terrified that our children would be swept by the current and our children would drown. The agents began to stab the inflatable raft. It was so inhumane the way we were treated by the U.S. agents. They knew about the risks and saw the children on the raft, but regardless they chose to flip the raft and they saw how desperate we became thinking our children were going to drown. They then threatened us, mocked us, and used obscene words.[37]

* * * *

THEORETICALLY THE policy was about COVID-19, but the actions on the ground ran against well-established public health guidelines. For example, it was well known that physical distancing could decrease the likelihood of the spread of the disease, but the migrants and asylum seekers crossing the southern border were detained in tightly confined and very cold places, like "ice boxes," remembers one migrant.[38] Another migrant recalled that despite the risk of spread of infection, they were not seen by anyone during their time in detention before being deported, even when they were coughing and visibly ill. "The conditions were bad [in detention], we were all sick, and we were in a room that was very cold and we got even more sick. We were not seen by a doctor, and we did not receive any medical attention."[39]

During the three-year period Title 42 remained in place, over 1.8 million expulsions were carried out, including people sent back to communities they had left because of persecution, torture, threats, and gender-based and gang violence.[40] Little to no correlation was found between immigrant entry and COVID-19 rates.[41] Furthermore, the conditions in migrant centers in Mexico soon started to deteriorate because of overcrowding, poor nutrition, dehydration, trauma, and anxiety.[42] Newborns and children were particularly affected by the policy that was widely decried by public health experts in the United States and around the world.[43]

News stories and pictures, including disturbing images of Haitian migrants being rounded up and poorly treated by border patrol on horses in Texas, gained national attention in September 2021, but the policy stayed in place for another year and a half.[44] During the first year, several aspects of the policy, including its application for unaccompanied minors, were challenged in various courts. As a result of these challenges, in November 2020, a federal judge ruled that unaccompanied minors cannot be sent back under the guise of Title 42.[45]

In the first year after winning the election, President Biden kept the policy in place, despite campaigning for a different policy.[46] The Biden administration continued to defend Title 42 restrictions and even argued in court that these expulsions were "necessary" in the light of "ongoing risks of transmission and spread of COVID-19."[47] Senior officials did, however, deflect when pressed on why the administration was keeping the policy in place. In October 2021, the secretary of the Department of Homeland Security (DHS) said that Title 42 was "not an immigration policy that we in this administration would embrace, but we view it as a public health imperative as the Centers for Disease Control has so ordered."[48] This was despite the fact that there was no consensus (and significant resistance) among senior CDC staff on whether Title 42 was necessary or even useful.[49] Lawyers, activists, public health experts, and clinicians continued to write, speak, and argue for ending a policy that was wrong. A letter signed by hundreds medical professionals and sent to the secretary of Health and Human Services and the CDC director noted that "the order does not protect Border Patrol agents, migrants or the American public from COVID-19.... Instead, your order reinforces a dehumanizing trope of migrants as vectors of disease."[50]

Eventually, the Biden administration announced that it would lift the Title 42 restrictions in May 2022, but the politicization of public health was not quite over as congressional members evaluated their own chances of reelection in light of the discussions on immigration in their districts.[51] In 2020, Senator Catherine Cortez Masto, a Democrat from Nevada, had signed a letter, along with other senators, that argued for ending Title 42, calling it a "CDC asylum ban."[52] By mid-2022, expecting stiff opposition to her reelection and recognizing that she had to court the conservative vote, she changed her position.[53] She joined a small group of Democratic senators who argued that rescinding Title 42 was "the wrong way" to address immigration and that it would "leave the administration unprepared for a surge at the border."[54] Eventually, the plan to lift the code had to be delayed for a year as courts reacted to lawsuits filed by several attorneys general from Republican-run states.[55] The states in support of keeping Title 42 argued that lifting the act would lead to an influx of migrants that would impose high costs on the states, including health care and education costs, and that the federal government had not considered these costs adequately. Title 42 was finally lifted in May 2023, and the long-term impact remains uncertain.[56]

What is perhaps important to recognize, and is consistent with other episodes in which real or perceived ideas about infection have been weaponized against outsiders, is that public health principles and clinical data did not support these actions. For Title 42 in particular, there was no support from the public health leadership of the country. The leadership of the National Institutes of Allergy and Infectious Diseases was clear in its assessment: "Focusing on immigrants, expelling them . . . is not the solution to an outbreak."[57] Other public health leaders, from a variety of academic institutions, were equally appalled by the policy.[58]

It is also important to note the exceptions that were made to Title 42 implementation, which uncover its political nature. In March 2022, in light of the Russia-Ukraine War, the Department of Homeland Security (DHS) issued a memo exempting Ukrainians from Title 42, stating,

> The Department of Homeland Security recognizes that the unjustified Russian war of aggression in Ukraine has created a humanitarian crisis. CBP is authorized, consistent with the Title 42 Order, on a case-by-case basis based on the totality of the circumstances, including considerations of humanitarian interests, to except Ukrainian nationals at land border ports of entry from Title 42. Non-citizens who are in possession of a valid Ukrainian passport or other valid Ukrainian identity document, and absent risk factors associated with national security or public safety, may be considered for exception from Title 42 under this guidance.[59]

The language making an exception for Ukrainian citizens and connecting it to war with Russia is particularly telling. No such exemption was made for Mexicans, Haitians, Hondurans, Guatemalans, or other communities from Central and South America, Asia, or Africa. While any group that is fleeing conflict and seeking safety deserves support, there are obvious unanswered questions about the DHS memo. Was there an assumption, by the government and DHS, that Ukrainians were somehow immune from the disease that poor communities from Central and South America were likely to bring to the United States? Or that the rules of public health surveillance applied differently if it was an adversary causing the displacement of people?

The selective application of the U.S. policy was not lost on me when I learned how the United States wanted Pakistan to act with regard to Afghans, who, desperate to seek safety, were showing up on Pakistan's borders.

In August 2021, U.S. troops and diplomatic staff abruptly left Afghanistan as Taliban forces gained ground and Afghan National Security Forces (ANSF) collapsed. U.S. and NATO forces evacuated only a small number of locals (a little over 120,000), most of whom were connected to the United States or the NATO mission in some way.[60] Large numbers of Afghans, who had no contacts or network, were equally desperate to leave.[61] Some wanted to flee because they were worried about an uncertain future under Taliban rule, especially if their political views and ideas did not align with the new regime's. Others because they felt that the coming months would bring greater food insecurity. These Afghans, with few possessions, tried to reach the borders with Iran and Pakistan and seek safety outside their country rather than go through another period of turmoil and chaos. The Pakistani government, because of its deep economic woes and widespread anti-Afghan sentiment in the country, had summarily said that it would not allow any more Afghan refugees into the country.[62] Pakistan had no political appetite for allowing more Afghans to come to the country. Many in Pakistan have long viewed Afghans as a menace and an ungrateful community that was bringing terrorism to the country and taking away precious resources that should only be for real Pakistanis.[63] Additionally, the pandemic was still going strong, and new variants were appearing routinely. Pakistan also has a poorly managed and underfunded public health system that was under tremendous stress.[64] COVID vaccines had just arrived a few months previously, and only a small fraction of the population had been inoculated. Distribution to small towns—including those close to the borders—was just starting in late summer 2021 and was not particularly effective.[65] Despite the vast differences between the capacity and strength of the public health systems in Pakistan and the United States, and knowing how Title 42 was being used in the United States to close its borders because of the pandemic, a senior State Department official had no qualms in saying in August 2021, "So, in a place like Pakistan, it'll be important that their borders remain open."[66] Unfortunately, no one asked the official why the same policy of keeping borders open could not apply to his own country.

10

Weaponizing the Shield

INFECTION AND BATTLEFRONT INJURIES HAVE
been intimately connected for as long as there have been wars.[1]
Wounds provide pathogens, which thrive in the soil and battlefields, a perfect entry into the body, where they have ample nour-
ishment to divide and spread. Some of the wounded die an
agonizing death from the ensuing infection; for others, it is the beginning of a lifelong disability. Nurses and doctors caring for
wounded soldiers knew the risks well, and even basic battlefield
hospitals have often focused on infection prevention with whatever
means were available at the time.[2] The availability of gun powder
created a new kind of war and caused injuries that resulted in depo-
sition of metal or organic matter inside the wound.[3] The infection
profile changed as a result of these new types of injuries, and so did
the practice of wartime care of soldiers. New practices in surgery
emerged along with greater care of the wound to control the spread
of infection.[4] The development of germ theory enabled military
physicians to use methods of extensive wound cleaning and removal of dead tissue when treating the wounded of the large global
conflicts of the early twentieth century, including World War I.
Doctors recognized that once bacterial infection sets in, it was very
difficult to control it without amputation: a process that was trau-
matic and that reduced the number of soldiers available for the
frontlines.[5] Anxiety about morbidity due to injury-related

infection also had a profound effect on the morale of recruits for these wars.

A lot changed in infection prevention and cure during the interwar years.[6] Driven in part by developments in chemistry and pharmacology, along with a better understanding of how bacteria multiplied in the enabling environment of wounds, new discoveries led to improved tools for controlling and treating infection, including isolation of infected patients and the use of antiseptic solutions for better wound care, along with new drugs (though still lacking broad efficacy) for managing some infections.[7]

A major breakthrough—the result of a sequence of chance encounters—was made in the lab of a bacteriologist named Alexander Fleming at St. Mary's Hospital in London.[8] In September 1928, after coming back from a vacation, Fleming noticed something unusual in one of the plates that was growing bacteria for his experiments. Fleming observed that fungus (which came from somewhere—perhaps a window or an open door) had come in contact with the bacteria on the plates. Instead of bacterial colonies, there was a clear ring around the mold on the plate indicating that the fungus had killed the bacteria. Fleming studied the fungus and determined that it was from the genus *Penicillium*. The active agent, with antibacterial properties in the fungus, that Fleming was able to extract was appropriately named *penicillin*. Fleming's early results showed that the new "drug" could potentially be useful against the particular bacteria (*staphylococci*) that cause staph infection. Fleming was a microbiologist, but he did not quite have the training in pharmacology and chemistry that was needed to take his discovery forward and convert it into a potent drug. It would take nearly a decade and a half for the transition from a lab discovery to the clinic to happen.

While penicillin was temporarily lost to the annals of academic papers, another class of antibiotic drugs was transforming infection control. Sulfonamide drugs (or *sulfa drugs* for short)—which were developed in the 1930s—were showing remarkable ability to fight bacterial infections.[9] As early as 1933, sulfa drugs had demonstrated efficacy in patients in European hospitals who were dying of septicemia (spread of infection in the blood stream).[10] Across the Atlantic, among those whose lives were saved by sulfa drugs (sold under the brand name Prontosil) was the young son of President Roosevelt, Franklin D. Roosevelt Jr., who had come down with a nasty infection. The unexpected recovery of FDR Jr. became national news. "When Franklin Roosevelt's throat grew swollen and raw and his temperature rose to a portentous degree, Dr. Tobey gave him hypodermic injections of Prontosil, made him swallow tablets of a modification named Prontylin. Under its influence, young Roosevelt rallied at once, thus providing an auspicious introduction for a product about which U.S. doctors and laymen have known little," wrote *Time* magazine.[11]

Sulfa drugs were an obvious choice during the early days of World War II as injuries at the front lines started to pile up in Europe. Since the drugs were widely available, both sides used them generously. There was, however, a troubling development. Over time, the drugs started to seem less effective against the infections they were earlier able to control, and by the early 1940s, it was clear that there was widespread "resistance," that is, the bacteria were no longer responding to the drugs.[12] The honeymoon period of sulfa drugs was coming to an abrupt end just as the injuries from war and the infections from those injuries were increasing sharply. Fortunately, in the waning days of sulfa drug efficacy, a new story—featuring an old antibiotic—was being written.[13]

Toward the end of the 1930s, a team of researchers at the Sir William Dunn School of Pathology in Oxford started studying penicillin and its effectiveness in combating infections.[14] Fleming's discovery from a decade ago was largely forgotten by then, and it is unclear exactly how and why the team at Oxford started to study penicillin. But the Oxford team was diverse in its training and had different expertise from Fleming's. They were able to extract penicillin from the mold and produce it in comparatively larger quantities than was possible a decade earlier. The team moved forward with animal tests and found the drug to be highly potent. In an experiment with eight mice infected with a virulent strain of *Streptococcus* (the bacterium that causes a variety of infections, including strep throat, pneumonia, and scarlet fever)—four were given penicillin and four were not. A day after the exposure to the bacteria, the four mice that were given penicillin were fine—the four that were not were all dead. The experimental result that was called a "miracle" (a term that would be used repeatedly in the years to come) was now ready for human trials.

The first human studies were conducted on an Oxford policeman, Albert Alexander, who had developed an infection a few weeks earlier that was oozing yellow pus.[15] An aggressive treatment with sulfa drugs was unable to control the spread of the infection, which had now reached his lungs. Penicillin purified by the Oxford team was used as a means of last resort. Alexander showed excellent progress within a day and was soon able to eat on his own. Penicillin had cleared the last hurdle—it was effective in humans and could be used to treat aggressive, life-threatening infections that were no longer treatable by sulfa drugs.

Scientists in the United Kingdom were convinced by the therapeutic potency of penicillin, but the methods to produce the drug in large quantities were hopeless. For example, the amount needed to treat just one adult patient like Alexander was nearly as much as all the reserves the Oxford team had. It became clear to the scientists at Oxford that the amount needed by a large group of people was not going to come from the laborious and complicated fermentation processes used by the UK researchers. Beyond the yield, the quality of the drug produced in British labs was also unsatisfactory. While the purity of the drug was vastly better than what Fleming had been able do in his lab, it was still only 5 percent pure. It was perhaps workable for a small set of clinical trials, but not at population scale. As Britain entered the war, and injuries, infection, and casualties started to mount, the need for effective treatment became even more acute. Both options for treating infection—a drug (sulfa) that was available in large quantities but was ineffective and one that was effective but scarce in the right doses—were dead ends. A better strategy was needed urgently.

The United States—given its financial and industrial resources—could provide respite at this stage.[16] Two British scientists from the Oxford team, Howard Florey and Norman Heatley, arrived in the United States in July 1941 to make their case to their U.S. counterparts for help in producing penicillin.[17] Florey had friends in influential research and government circles in the country, and his contacts led them to the Northern Regional Research Laboratory (NRRL) of the U.S. Department of Agriculture in Peoria, Illinois, with the hope that the national lab infrastructure could help the British team improve drug quality and yield.[18] The NRRL team requested samples of mold from around the world, searching for a strain of fungus that would produce more penicillin in a shorter time. The successful candidate came not from an exotic location in a distant land but from a fruit seller close to home: a rotten cantaloupe from a fruit market near Peoria became the source of the desired strain.[19] The moldy fruit produced at least two hundred times more penicillin than did the species of mold Fleming had worked with.[20] Further refinement led to another fivefold increase.[21]

Alongside a better strain to produce penicillin was improvement in fermentation methods. The impact of the merger between a better strain and improved technology for growing the source of the drug (a process called *deep tank fermentation*) was dramatic.[22] The U.S. government's next step was to engage large pharmaceutical companies like Pfizer and Merck to scale production.[23] A meeting in October 1941 with the Committee on Medical Research (CMR), the Office of Scientific Research and Development (OSRD), and senior executives from several pharmaceutical companies placed penicillin production at the top of its agenda.[24] While the issue of drug production was serious and somewhat urgent, it was to become an issue of highest priority in just a few weeks with the attack on Pearl Harbor on December 7, 1941.[25]

* * * *

OVER THE COURSE of the following two years, partnerships between several arms of the U.S. government, including the Department of Agriculture (USDA), and pharmaceutical companies unlocked millions of dollars of research and development funds.[26] The results were phenomenal. At the end of 1941, the United States did not have enough penicillin to treat a single patient.[27] By the end of 1942, the quantities available were sufficient for approximately a hundred patients.[28] By September 1943, there was enough penicillin to satisfy the demand of not just the U.S. military but all the Allied Forces.[29] For the D-Day landing, 2.3 million doses were manufactured.[30] In August 1944, *Life Magazine* had an advertisement from a pharmaceutical company with an image of two soldiers—one was injured and the other was treating the injured combatant. The poster read "Thanks to Penicillin . . . He will Come Home!"[31] Another wartime poster described penicillin as a shield protecting the brave men at the front from enemy fire.[32] By the end of the war, the United States was producing well above 6 billion units of penicillin. There is broad agreement among analysts and military historians that penicillin played a direct role in turning the tide of the war in favor of the Allies—not just in terms of saving lives and preventing infection but also indirectly by boosting the morale of the troops. The death rate from bacterial pneumonia, just one of the infections faced by the troops, for example, was 18 percent during World War I. It was less than 1 percent in World War II.[33] The remarkable success of penicillin was not simply because of a strain from a rotten cantaloupe but also because of the direct involvement of the U.S. military and the resources it made available. During the second half of the war, the U.S. high command had put penicillin production as the second-highest priority, only behind the Manhattan Project.[34]

The story of antibiotics is often viewed in stages. It starts from the process of discovery dating back to the dawn of germ theory and the ideas proposed in the early part of the twentieth century about "magic bullets" that would disarm the pathogen but leave the healthy cells unscathed. And it follows with the accidental discovery of penicillin, the rise of sulfa drugs in the 1930s and their rapid decline, the global domination of commercially available penicillin starting in the early 1940s, and the golden era of antibiotics that continued for nearly two decades after the war with new and ever more powerful drugs appearing on the market.[35] There were strong signs that nature—in particular, rich soil—could be tapped for new sources of antibiotics. Clinicians and the public had a high demand for antibiotics, and of course there was good money to be made.[36] Soon after the war, entire divisions in pharmaceutical companies were making new drugs and working (sometimes in ethically dubious ways) with willing clinicians who were prescribing them generously and without recognizing the real dangers of drug resistance.[37] A sense of invincibility against nasty bugs prevailed. Though there were strong early indications of rapid development and proliferation of resistance, it was largely ignored as there were always newer and more potent drugs on the market. This honeymoon period did not last forever, and it led to the current situation we find ourselves in, where antimicrobial resistance is among the most serious global health threats of our time.

The intermediate and honeymoon period of antibiotics is important not only because of the excesses that came with a misguided sense that there was a seemingly inexhaustible source of new drugs but also because of the new way of thinking that emerged about infectious diseases and who should have access to their cures. The United States and the Allied Forces saw the extraordinary power of antibiotics—one that went well beyond the needs on the battlefield. Countries around the world did too. But the world was once again split. During the Cold War, the United States and its allies (in particular Britain) felt that access to antibiotics was somehow the right only of those living in the *free world* (as opposed to those in Communist countries).[38] In 1949, the United States created an embargo that blocked any material of strategic importance from being sent to countries in the Soviet bloc.[39] Antibiotics were part of these strategically important materials.

By this time, the patents on how to produce penicillin were in the public domain and antibiotics could be produced anywhere— but the equipment necessary for the process was largely in the hands of the United States and the United Kingdom.[40] In the absence of appropriate equipment, countries in the Soviet bloc could not produce either the desired quantities of penicillin or drugs of acceptable quality. The need—however—continued to grow so much that the World Health Organization in March 1949 tried to intervene and buy equipment from the United States to enable the poorer countries of Eastern Europe to produce penicillin for their sick citizens. Poland, Czechoslovakia, and Yugoslavia had complained to the WHO that their effort to combat and treat venereal diseases was severely hampered by their inability to produce antibiotics. With a mandate to help and provide relief to a large number of displaced persons during and after World War II, the United National Refugee and Relief Administration (UNRRA) established drug production plants in Poland and Czechoslovakia for making penicillin—but the key equipment and its spare parts were manufactured exclusively in the United States. When the WHO brought up the issue in a meeting, the U.S. representative responded that the discussion on equipment and parts for making lifesaving drugs was not appropriate for the WHO.[41] In 1949, when the issue of lifting the embargo on the equipment necessary for efficient penicillin manufacture came up, the UK Defense and Foreign Office resisted, saying that keeping the embargo on the equipment was of "extreme importance from the point of view of bacteriological warfare."[42] The CIA was also actively looking at the manufacture of antibiotics in the USSR and its allies. A detailed 1954 report from the CIA is quite telling, where, as historian

Mauro Capocci notes, CIA officers took pride in showing that "US exports of antibiotics to the Soviet Bloc dwindled from a substantial $12,388,000 in 1950 to a mere $4,000 in 1952."[43]

* * * *

ANTIBIOTICS CONTINUED TO be a major topic of discussion at the highest levels of the U.S. government, including at the National Security Council (NSC). The issue of antibiotics and the embargo came up several times in an NSC meeting on November 5, 1953, that was presided over by President Eisenhower and attended by the secretaries of defense and state, as well as military leadership.[44] The meeting minutes describe how antibiotics—which were desperately needed by China—were viewed as a political and diplomatic tool as described in a conversation between Assistant Secretary of State for Commerce and International Affairs Samuel Anderson and Under Secretary of State Walter Smith. The minutes note that

> Secretary Anderson then offered to illustrate the general point of the need for reviewing our stringent prohibition of trade with Communist China by special reference to antibiotics. If, said Secretary Anderson, we were prepared to loosen up on trade in these items, which the Chinese were desperately anxious to obtain and which our allies were anxious to sell them, it might result in our being able to induce our allies to restrict more effectively their trade with Communist China on items of genuine strategic importance. On the whole, this exchange, said Secretary Anderson, had much to recommend it in terms of the genuine advantage to the United States. To this argument Secretary Smith added that the State Department was now very greatly concerned over the humanitarian aspect of our embargo on antibiotics. Now that the actual fighting in Korea had ended, the United States was going to be very hard pressed to withstand propaganda that it was deliberately withholding needed drugs from China.[45]

This discussion referred to the situation during the Korean war, when the drugs were considered an essential material in the military campaign and hence viewed from a lens of national security rather than as a lifesaving commodity. It was only after the Korean armistice in 1953 that the embargo on the antibiotics was finally lifted.[46]

* * * *

THE POTENCY OF antibiotics and the anxiety about bacterial warfare allowed for new ideas to emerge among military strategists and physicians working with them. These ideas focused not just on defense against deadly pathogens but also on using this defensive shield to create more potent weapons that would not respond to frontline antibiotics. For example, questions were asked about the limits of antibiotics.[47] Could there be weapons that would cause disease that no antibiotics could treat? What would that weapon look like? How would it be developed and deployed? This was far from the original and continued mission of antibiotic discovery but inevitable in the climate of *us versus them*, and an inevitable consequence of the thinking that did not find the destruction of civilian infrastructure in the case of war problematic.

Antibiotics became part and parcel of developing biological weapons (discussed in the previous chapter). The efficacy of biological weapons was intimately connected to whether an antibiotic would be effective, as the goal of the weapons program was to create new pathogens that could evade the shield provided by antibiotics. New weapons could not be produced if it was not for the availability of antibiotics that—despite their promise in saving countless lives—acted as a fuel for the production of tools of mass destruction. As more potent antibiotics became available, the limits of their potency became the starting point of the destructive power of new biological weapons.

The interconnected world of privilege and potent medicines is not simply a feature of war and weapons. In times of crisis, essential drugs and vaccines have been influenced by market forces that favor the privileged while denying care to those who lack power or resources. For example, during the COVID-19 pandemic, rich countries bought stocks of vaccines that amounted to more than their entire population while the poorest countries did not even have a fraction of the vaccines needed for their population.[48] When the first vaccines were rolled out, rich countries bought essentially all current and future supplies of the vaccines. In November 2021, it was reported that while 65 percent of the population in wealthy countries were able to be vaccinated, in some of the poorest countries on the planet less than 3 percent of the population could get the vaccine.[49]

When vaccines were finally available in larger quantities—they were often of little use to the poorest countries. In January 2022, it was reported that poorer nations rejected nearly 100 million doses of COVID-19 vaccines because they were about to expire.[50] It is not hard to imagine that vaccines close to their expiration date would never be sent to richer and more influential countries. The inequity hit the low-income countries hard, where their populations suffered because of the lack of vaccines and adequate treatment.[51]

In the time of acute crisis, governments used vaccine diplomacy—a rather polite term for *global competition*—to increase their influence in low-income countries. The United States, countries in the European Union, Russia, China, and India all vied for global influence in countries that could be cashed in later.

In this new competition, countries like the United States told allies, such as Brazil, to reject vaccines made by Russia. As discussed earlier, the United States also launched a misinformation campaign against its Chinese competitors, who were providing WHO-approved vaccines to dozens of low- and middle-income countries.[52]

Lifesaving commodities and technologies to prevent and treat infection—from drugs to vaccines—are often not viewed as a common good by rich and powerful countries. Instead, they are commodities that are used for specific political purposes, including building relationships with some nations and undermining the efforts of others. Having an embargo on antibiotics to countries that desperately need them to save the lives of the sick and the vulnerable, when there is a surplus and ample capacity to produce more, is similar to hoarding surplus food during a bumper crop season while there is a famine in a country that wants it and is willing to pay for it. But a country may refuse to give them food just because it may not like their government—or because it does not believe that the lives of the people in those countries are worth saving.

Conclusion
Ending the Exploitation Enterprise

IN NORTHWEST PAKISTAN, A COUPLE OF HOURS drive from the home where I grew up, many people are scarred by the CIA vaccination campaign. These scars are both physical and emotional. There are disabled young men and women who missed their polio vaccines, after the local tribal leaders threatened the polio workers, and many others who lost their family members in the various attacks on health workers that were carried out in the region in the last decade. As I listened to their stories while doing research for this book, I wondered: Why should these people, or anyone for that matter, have to pay the price of a scheme concocted thousands of miles away for a political goal that had nothing to do with them in the first place? Stories of people like the ones I heard in Pakistan drove me to learn about how infection treatment and research can be weaponized and exploited.

* * * *

JUST AS THERE are many with emotional trauma in the country that I grew up in, plenty carry deep scars of neglect and apathy in the country I live in now. These scars reflect a parallel dimension of how we deal with infectious diseases—an impulsive response that blames the victim and their morality for the pain they face and shuts down any serious discussion on how to help. It is a story of deliberate inaction that has caused suffering among those who were desperately in need of care.

During the 1980s, when the first reports of HIV became public, the reaction from the government and its supporters was not one of empathy or concern. It was rooted in ignorance, denial, and victim-blaming. In the years that followed, thousands paid dearly as a result of this attitude, many with their lives, others through a miserable existence.

The first reports of HIV in the United States came in the summer of 1981 when the Centers for Disease Control and Prevention reported rare lung infections in previously healthy gay men in Los Angeles.[1] Soon, reports followed of rare and opportunistic infections in other parts of the country.[2] It became clear that mortality in many of these patients was caused by their immune system failing and no longer able to fight disease. By the end of 1981, 337 cases of this new illness were reported—out of which 130 (38 percent) died not long after their initial diagnosis.[3] Because the disease was seen largely in homosexual men—it was referred to in public by various terms that included "gay plague" or "gay-related immune deficiency" (GID—a term used by newspapers, including the *New York Times*, at the time).[4] Unsurprisingly, the reaction from various quarters was to blame the disease on the patients' immoral behavior and see it as a punishment for their own actions.

* * * *

IN SEPTEMBER 1982, the CDC used the term *AIDS*—Acquired Immune Deficiency Syndrome—for the first time and defined it as "a disease at least moderately predictive of a defect in cell-mediated immunity occurring in a person with no known cause for diminished resistance to that disease."[5] Despite this, the White House (and the press pool covering the White House) continued to call it the gay plague. One particular exchange (reported by *Vanity Fair* in 2015), using archival audio recording from October 1982 between White House press secretary Larry Speakes and journalist Lester Kinsolving, is particularly telling:[6]

> LESTER KINSOLVING: Does the president have any reaction to the
> announcement by the Centers for Disease Control in Atlanta
> that AIDS is now an epidemic in over 600 cases?
> LARRY SPEAKES: AIDS? I haven't got anything on it.
> LESTER KINSOLVING: Over a third of them have died. It's known
> as "gay plague." [Press pool laughter] No, it is. It's a pretty serious thing. One in every three people that get this have died. And
> I wonder if the president was aware of this.
> LARRY SPEAKES: I don't have it. [Press pool laughter] Do you?
> LESTER KINSOLVING: You don't have it? Well I'm relieved to hear
> that, Larry! [Press pool laughter]
> LARRY SPEAKES: Do you?
> LESTER KINSOLVING: No, I don't.
> LARRY SPEAKES: You didn't answer my question. How do you
> know? [Press pool laughter.]
> LESTER KINSOLVING: Does the president—in other words the
> White House—look on this as a great joke?
> LARRY SPEAKES: No, I don't know anything about it, Lester.

By this time in 1982, over 850 people in the United States had died from AIDS.[7]

As the number of those who were suffering increased and pressure mounted from several public health researchers and physicians, the Reagan administration made a series of empty promises about AIDS being a high priority but failed to mobilize the necessary financial resources to tackle the challenge. In August 1983, Dr. Marcus Conant, a prominent physician who was treating AIDS patients in California, told the House Oversight Subcommittee on AIDS that "the failure to respond to this epidemic now borders on a national scandal. The second point is that this body, Congress and indeed the American people have been misled about the response.

We have been led to believe that the response has been timely and that the response has been appropriate, and I would suggest to you that is not correct."[8]

The Reagan administration's response continued to be weak well into 1984, when over 4,000 people in the United States had died from AIDS.[9] During another press conference, Larry Speakes once again continued to make light of the situation in an exchange with Lester Kinsolving. Here is an excerpt from the audio clip from 1984:[10]

LESTER KINSOLVING: Since the Centers for Disease Control in Atlanta report is going to ... [*Press pool laughter*]

LARRY SPEAKES: This is going to be an AIDS question.

LESTER KINSOLVING: ... that an estimated ...

LARRY SPEAKES: You were close.

LESTER KINSOLVING: Can I ask the question, Larry? That an estimated 300,000 people have been exposed to AIDS, which can be transmitted through saliva. Will the president as commander-in-chief take steps to protect armed forces' food and medical services from AIDS patients or those who run the risk of spreading AIDS in the same manner that they ban typhoid fever people from being involved in the health or food services?

LARRY SPEAKES: I don't know.

LESTER KINSOLVING: Is the president concerned about this subject, Larry?

LARRY SPEAKES: I haven't heard him express concern.

LESTER KINSOLVING: That seems to have evoked such jocular reaction here. [*Press pool laughter*]

UNIDENTIFIED PERSON: It isn't only the jocks, Lester.

UNIDENTIFIED PERSON: Has he sworn off water faucets now?

LESTER KINSOLVING: No, but I mean is he going to do anything, Larry?

LARRY SPEAKES: Lester, I have not heard him express anything. Sorry.

LESTER KINSOLVING: You mean he has expressed no opinion about this epidemic?

LARRY SPEAKES: No, but I must confess I haven't asked him about it.

LESTER KINSOLVING: Will you ask him, Larry?

LARRY SPEAKES: Have you been checked? [*Press pool laughter*]

UNIDENTIFIED PERSON: Is the president going to ban mouth-to-mouth kissing?

LESTER KINSOLVING: What? Pardon? I didn't hear your answer.

LARRY SPEAKES: [*Laughs*] Ah, it's hard work. I don't get paid enough. Um. Is there anything else we need to do here?

Outside the White House, prominent groups that had supported Reagan's conservative agenda were also unhappy that he was even considering federal funding for providing treatment for gay people. For example, in 1983 the vice president of the Moral Majority (founded by Baptist minister Jerry Falwell Sr. in 1977 to promote conservative causes), an organization that had strongly supported Reagan's election, said, "We feel the deepest sympathy for AIDS victims but I'm upset that the government is not spending money to protect the general public from the gay plague. What I see is a commitment to spend our tax dollars on research to allow these diseased homosexuals to go back to their perverted practices without any standards of accountability."[11]

* * *

BEYOND THE ATTITUDES of the Reagan administration and the groups that were promoting conservative causes, the attitudes in the U.S. Congress were also making research and treatment of HIV patients difficult. For example, Congressman Henry Waxman, who had tried to increase funding for research and treatment, found strong opposition from his colleagues, including Congressman Bill Dannemeyer from California and Dan Burton from Indiana. As Waxman recalled in his memoirs, "When Dannemeyer weighed in, his determined priority was not research or prevention, but rather rounding up gay men and quarantining them on an island in the South Pacific, a proposal he called a press conference to announce."[12] Similarly, it was reported in newspapers that Dan Burton had stopped eating soup because he believed that a waiter might have AIDS and give it to him by coming in contact with his meal.[13] The stigmatization of homosexual persons was seen across party lines. Florida Democratic senator Lawton Chiles famously said, "I guess you can say that as long as this disease is confined among homosexuals no real danger."[14]

Continued reports that HIV was largely present among homosexual men, or transmitted through needles reused for drug injection, made strong action politically unappealing. Since the communities that were impacted were either stigmatized or socioeconomically disadvantaged, the disease remained a low priority despite its mounting death toll.

At the same time, Dr. David Purcell (who worked at the Division of HIV/AIDS Prevention, Centers for Disease Control and Prevention) noted the impact on the lives of people who had AIDS and how society treated them. "People with AIDS were kicked out of homes by family members and landlords, not touched or avoided by medical professionals, and lost their jobs. Obituaries often excluded AIDS as the cause of death, and surviving partners were often not named as bereaved survivors or able to obtain survivors benefits," he wrote in a paper in 2021 commemorating the fortieth anniversary of the reporting of the first case in 1981.[15] President Reagan mentioned AIDS for the first time in 1985 in a press conference.[16] His first speech on the topic was not delivered until 1987.[17] By that time, over 14,000 people had died of HIV in the United States.[18]

Over the last three decades, fortunately, the situation around HIV has improved in terms of diagnosis, treatment, and management of the disease. Today there are approximately 1.2 million people living with HIV in the United States, and many are able to manage the disease as a chronic condition.[19] Research funding, which has increased substantially since the early days of HIV in the United States, has resulted in new discoveries that have paved the way for better diagnostics and improved therapeutics.[20] Consequently, the likelihood of surviving beyond a few months or a year after testing positive for HIV has increased dramatically. The credit for this extraordinary achievement goes not only to lab scientists and physicians but also to community organizers, social workers, and concerned citizens. Social activists and community support groups that first emerged in the 1980s have continued to play a strong role in generating public awareness, tackling stigmas, improving access to care, and forcing large pharmaceutical companies to change their practices so that communities in places like sub-Saharan Africa could afford lifesaving drugs.[21]

Despite major gains, racial and socioeconomic disparity continues to be intertwined with HIV in the United States.[22] Black Americans, despite making up approximately 12 percent of the total population, make up over 40 percent of all HIV infections and 44 percent of all deaths from HIV. Similarly, Hispanic and Latino communities make up approximately 18 percent of the total population but account for 25 percent of HIV-infected persons. Stigmatization, poverty, and lack of access to care determine not just the likelihood of getting HIV but also who gets to have appropriate and affordable care and who gets to live with dignity and who does not.

In the grand scheme of infection and its impact on disadvantaged groups, HIV has similarities to other diseases where victim-blaming (e.g., cholera) and perceptions of immorality (syphilis) shaped the public narrative about the disease. But it also presents another dimension of why an infectious disease destroyed the lives of those who could have been saved or at least cared for with dignity in their most painful moments. Here, the situation was not active government intent or policy to target a particular group (for example, development of biological weapons, testing of hypothesis about gonorrhea on inmates, or denial of asylum) but deliberate inaction driven by apathy and politics despite the urgent need and repeated pleading by activists, scientists, clinicians, and public health experts. The availability or denial of care based on how someone looks or whether someone does or does not conform to some set of social values continues to define who gets to be treated when sick and who does not.

* * * *

THE QUESTIONS IN this book go beyond the basic science of infectious disease. We cannot extricate scientific research from the enterprise of exploitation. We should ask: Why does infection continue to be weaponized for political purposes? How can we ensure that we stop this exploitation? To answer these questions, we have to first understand the science of infection, give scholars of infectious disease the resources to investigate and the ability to share their findings freely (especially when they challenge our existing notions and policies), give the evidence about disease the due attention it deserves, embrace ambiguity when we do not know, and ensure that our views are not clouded by political expediencies or racial prejudices. At the same time, we need to take a broader and holistic look at who is impacted by infectious diseases and our research approach? We need to look at the political motives of countries, institutions, and the individuals who set these goals and how institutions view vulnerable individuals and consider them less deserving of care and support. The goals that facilitate the weaponization of infection may be associated with national security or defense; a desire to keep the population homogeneous; a distrust of other races; an opportunity to exact revenge on a group that is disliked for racial, ethnic, or religious reasons; or a worldview that sees exploitation as a necessary cost for greater scientific progress and the accumulation of beneficial knowledge.

On the face of it, some of these goals may seem independent, perhaps even contradictory, of each other, but they all are part of a world where knowledge is ripe for abuse. Knowledge of infection—or the research to seek that knowledge about infectious diseases—is potent because it exists in two worlds: the real world, where there are bacteria, viruses, and parasites that cause disease, disability, and suffering; and the world of our imagination, where the idea of infection influences our thoughts, anxieties, and actions. The movement between these two worlds makes infection a unique weapon in the hands of people and institutions who may not share the values of dignity for every person, without discrimination.

Infection, on its own, does not stop Black sharecroppers in Alabama from getting penicillin for syphilis—and allows them to suffer for forty years. That required deliberations in conferences and enactment of active barriers so the patients could not access the care they needed and deserved. And infection does not make an otherwise healthy population in the urban centers of the Soviet Union become incapable of doing basic daily tasks. That required a military leadership that wanted to construct biological weapons to harm citizens who live in enemy territory. Exploiting vulnerable people requires a motive and an associated bureaucratic process to enact that motive. It requires real people, in positions of power and authority, to come up with an idea and real people to work alongside them to operationalize the idea in the layers of the system. And finally, it requires the support of those in the highest offices to ensure the continuity and sustainability of the mission that originated from that idea.

It is perhaps easy to dismiss those who craft these ideas as racist. Some may have those traits, but it would be naïve and grossly inaccurate to assume that everyone who has been directly, or indirectly, involved in policies and studies that inflicted harm on others in the name of infectious disease research or in the creation of biological weapons for national security is motivated by the same emotions or reason. As hard as it may be to imagine that those who take their Hippocratic oath seriously could be involved in creating biological weapons or could be comfortable with supporting a study of exposing incarcerated or mentally unwell persons in another country to gonorrhea, we know that there have been plenty of distinguished and well-regarded clinicians who were involved in these projects and studies. While some attended schools with a long history of training doctors who believed in eugenics, many others had otherwise extraordinary careers as public health professionals, advocated for improved access to medicines, confronted stigmas around infections, substantially improved public awareness through their writings and speeches, successfully lobbied Congress for increased funding for community health programs for disease prevention, and led distinguished careers as scholars, scientists, and research administrators.

Likewise, not everyone who was involved was a clinician or a politician driven by a particular ideology. Many were lab-based scientists interested in studying fundamental biological processes— engineers, chemists, physicists, and mathematicians who contributed to the exploitation enterprise in some way or the other. From a strict sense, these people were not bound by the Hippocratic oath. But should they not have seen what their work was being used for and what it was doing to individuals and communities? The absence of a Hippocratic oath should not mean the omission of the ethical analysis of actions and policies whatsoever. For example, how could a forty-year-long study denying care to an impoverished community be justified, not once, but during repeated discussions of the study? How could anyone argue that total wars required the complete annihilation of the enemy, and this meant harming unarmed, unsuspecting, and innocent citizens including babies and children?

While human motives are often complicated, we do have some evidence from the personal papers, diaries, testimonies, and interviews of those who led, supported, or participated in various studies and projects. We also have evidence of how researchers and scholars who worked on these projects for the state and its institutions benefited from state support in the form of grants and awards. Furthermore, national defense, particularly during times of active conflict or after a terrorist incident, has often enabled people to let their guard down and disregard ethical principles. The heat of these moments has resulted in them prioritizing some lives over others to the extent that they can no longer hear the screams of innocent children being bombarded. The idea of self-preservation, or the argument of national security, is easy to exploit, and voices of reason, concern, and humanity are usually silenced (often aggressively and with wide public support) at those times.

Similarly, scientists and researchers often concern themselves with the immediate and actively disconnect themselves from the consequences of their actions. In hindsight, it is very easy to connect the research with the exploitation of that research, but at that particular moment, research scholars tend to focus on the particular experiment, the specific data set, and fail to recognize how their research is being used. The attraction of funding and recognition further increases this myopia.

The episodes discussed in this book are all in the past. There is some reason to be hopeful knowing that the Tuskegee experiment was discontinued, the biological weapons program has ended, HIV care is more accessible than it was in the 1980s, and Title 42 restrictions were lifted after three years. But that sense of optimism needs to be tempered by acknowledging that new political and geopolitical realities will create new avenues of weaponization, fueled in part by new discoveries. There are legitimate concerns about how new technologies, such as artificial intelligence, are likely to increase the marginalization of vulnerable groups. Similarly, drones are being used to deter migrants from seeking asylum, digital technologies are being employed to exclude stateless persons from accessing health care services, and biometric systems are being employed to share the data of at-risk communities with authorities across the world who have no concern for their safety or well-being. There is ample reason for us to be cautious and to question our euphoria about the next big breakthrough.[23]

* * * *

JUST AS WE reflect on the harm committed in the name of national security or scientific research, we should also look at what has worked as we come up with a prescription for a better future. Though many clinicians and medical researchers have been involved in the multiple episodes discussed in this book, by and large, most doctors and physician researchers uphold the values of the Hippocratic oath and think carefully about the "do no harm" part of that pledge. That question of harm, however, cannot simply be viewed in a narrow patient-doctor relationship but must extend to all aspects of research that can touch the lives of people well beyond the experiences of an individual clinician and the patient (or subject) in the study. Also, no such oath exists for physicists, chemists, mathematicians, biomedical engineers, or political scientists. It would be naïve to imagine that we can create Hippocratic oaths in all disciplines, but we should think about why the Hippocratic oath works (most of the time) and how to incorporate principles of personal responsibility and accountability as we train these professionals. This would require a deeper understanding of how we teach about human lives and values, rights and privileges, and accountability of our actions. I am painfully aware of how far we are from where we ought to be. Most of my students—including those who are well read beyond their disciplines—have never heard of the Tuskegee study or the U.S. biological weapons program, and almost none know about the CIA's vaccination campaign in Pakistan. The onus for that is on me and my colleagues.

Lessons from the painful history of technology, infection, and exploitation tell us how some of these programs ended. For example, when it came to the Tuskegee study, it was the work of individuals within government institutions (e.g., Peter Buxtun), journalists

(Jean Heller), and others who saw the programs for what they were. Scholars like Susan Reverby brought the horrors of the Guatemala study to public attention. Similarly, thousands of activists all over the world took to the streets and forced their governments to change course, take HIV seriously, and provide better care for patients all over the world. It is also important to remember that these efforts took years. Additionally, projects that seemed to end with a single executive order (for example, President Nixon's declaration ending the biological weapons program, President Obama's decision to stop the use of vaccination campaigns to gather intelligence, and President Biden's lifting of the COVID-19-era Title 42 restrictions) rested on the efforts of countless people, in offices large and small, and in communities all across the country and around the world, who worked tirelessly for years before they saw the results.

The lesson for us who have benefited from a better world is to recognize the sacrifice of individuals, both within and outside government circles, who risked their lives and careers to speak the truth. Most importantly, we need to rethink, as a society, how to view scientific research and advancement and not shy away from discussing the ethical implications of scientific advancement, especially on communities that have been historically marginalized. While strongly supporting scientific research, including basic research that may not seem to have a direct impact immediately, we must also recognize that discoveries need proactive (and not reactive) guardrails to protect the vulnerable, whether in development of technologies or in their broad rollout. Ethics cannot simply be an afterthought or a reactive impulse. Our understanding of how someone may be harmed by development, testing, or implementation of new technology has to go beyond the performative aspects of consent and has to be viewed in terms of potential future impact. These ethical guardrails must be universal, not territorial. What is an unacceptable use of a discovery for citizens in the United States should be unacceptable for everyone else, whether they live in an exclusive neighborhood and affluent gated communities or in a refugee camp. This may seem difficult—or perhaps impossible—in a world where international cooperation has become more difficult, but our principles should not be dependent on the political alliances of a particular moment in time. International institutional solidarity is weak and fragmented at the moment, but international *human* solidarity, particularly among the young generation, is strong and continues to inspire.

There is reason to believe that people in different nations care about one another and stand up for one another's rights, even when countries and institutions are highly suspicious of each other. For example, today, global public sentiment and potential outrage would force countries to think twice before developing—or worse, deploying—biological weapons. This was not the case during most of the twentieth century. This sense of care and concern for all should not just be a slogan but should be a core principle as we develop and deploy technologies. Here, it is important to make the distinction between discovery, which is often serendipitous, and technology development, which is deliberate. While supporting greater opportunities for discovery, with important checks to ensure that the principle of do no harm, to anyone, even in research, we should also demand greater scrutiny for technology development and deployment.

Infectious disease research—like many other branches of science—has to be cognizant of two opposing forces of exploitation. The first is those whose own knowledge of science may be lacking and see the scientific enterprise as an evil empire, or may have a personal agenda, thereby concocting conspiracy theories that do immense harm. These theories find fertile ground during times of distress (pandemics, humanitarian crises, etc.) and among those who have other reasons to be skeptical of government or private sector institutions. The other group that one needs to guard against is one that is not skeptical of science or unfamiliar with the results of research but is uninterested in ensuring that everyone benefits equally or is not bothered by the misuse of good science for political purposes. Both of these groups undermine the foundations of honest research—and in a strange way, reinforce each other. The public trust is undermined—and conspiracy theories take hold—when good science is hijacked for political purposes. The broader anti-vaccination sentiment in Pakistan, including the refusal for polio vaccination in rural areas of the country, has been influenced by the CIA campaign discussed in this book. Similarly, data from COVID-19 vaccination rates across the country has shown that the long shadow of the Tuskegee study continues to shape how Black communities view vaccination drives. As one recent study on disparity in COVID-19 vaccination among white and Black Americans (especially around Tuskegee) noted, "The lingering mistrust stemming from the Tuskegee Study has contributed to unequal vaccination rates between African Americans and the rest of America."[24]

Tackling mistrust—and concurrently misinformation—will require an emphasis on sound science, transparency, and ethics that makes it morally reprehensible and legally impossible for scientific discoveries to be used to harm anyone and for the scientific process to be up for robust critique that it does not disregard the human dignity of any group—no matter their racial makeup or socioeconomic standing. I recognize that this is easier said than done, but this is the only solution, not just because it is morally right but also because it is necessary to preserve the global public trust in science and the profound power of its solutions for our collective welfare. This requires opportunities to reflect through curricula in science and engineering, medicine and public health. Science and medicine curriculum, at all levels, cannot be focused solely on the technical while ignoring how good science has been used to harm others. The inspiring stories about the process of discovery, which are absolutely essential, need to connect with the instances on how those discoveries have been used—both for human welfare and for human suffering. In order for us to imagine a better future, we have to face our own past and simultaneously be proud of the incredible achievements in science, engineering, and medicine and acknowledge our serious failings.

There will likely be new technologies and discoveries in the years to come that are beyond our imagination. Many of these will provide extraordinary opportunities to save lives and improve our well-being; some will be ripe for exploitation for political purposes. The only way to minimize this risk is to fight against the dehumanization of individuals. It is when we think of others as enemies, as uncivilized, as inferior or expendable, we convince ourselves that our actions are not only justified but essential. We must always resist that urge.

Acknowledgments

The world changed as I was working on this book. Infection shaped our world, and solutions rooted in infectious disease research saved the lives of hundreds of millions of people in all parts of the world. At the same time, misinformation and conspiracy theories found new champions. These voices were multiplied by social media. Some of these movements have now become mainstream and are likely to have a profound effect on the health of people—especially those who may already be struggling because of poverty, injustice, or lack of adequate care. In the midst of this confusion and misinformation, talking about how infectious disease research can be weaponized for political purposes is a difficult task. How does one defend scientific method and discovery and believe that the world is healthier and safer because of vaccines and therapeutics but also acknowledge the unimaginable harm inflicted in Tuskegee and Guatemala, all in the name of studying disease and saving lives? As I grappled with these questions, many of which are discussed in the book, I benefited from the wisdom, advice, and support of many people who guided me, helped me think through the issues, and challenged my assumptions. Some of these people are trusted colleagues and old friends; others, complete strangers. Some lived close to home, and others in villages and small towns thousands of miles away. Some I mention by name; others prefer to remain anonymous for a variety of reasons. Their generosity during my research, fieldwork, and writing stages not only made this book possible but also left a permanent imprint on me. I am indebted to all of them.

I was extremely fortunate to have Nisrine Rahmaoui as my research assistant during the formative stages of research and writing. Nisrine, an undergraduate student at Boston University, was an exemplary colleague. She was thoughtful, rigorous, hardworking, and always eager to learn. She was well read and very attentive to details. Above all, she was always cheerful. Given the pandemic restrictions, most of my interactions with her were on Zoom or via email, yet her enthusiasm, kindness, and optimism were infectious. I am deeply grateful to her for the work she did on the book and for the light she brought into the lives of everyone around her. During the later stages of writing and proofreading, two other colleagues, Helen Lindsay and Rana Hussein, carefully read the manuscript and helped with the meticulous task of checking references. I am honored to have them as my trusted colleagues.

During the research and writing process, I would sometimes get stuck, or would come across something that did not quite make sense. Friends, colleagues, and mentors were there to show the path forward. Professor Susan Reverby, at Wellesley College, was generous with her time and instrumental in helping me understand the history and politics at the core of syphilis studies, those in the United States and abroad. Students and fellows in my research group were always there to help me sharpen my arguments or encourage me to reconsider my thesis. I am grateful to them for their unwavering support.

I have the privilege of working with some of the most decent and thoughtful people at the Center on Forced Displacement. Their commitment to human dignity inspires me every day. Professor Carrie Preston is not just a colleague at the center and a close friend, she is also a mentor who has shaped my teaching and writing. I benefited tremendously from her encouragement and wise counsel. Generous financial support from the Schooner Foundation for my research made the book possible.

The journey of this book was also shepherded by Michelle Tessler, my literary agent, and Ben Woodward, my editor at The New Press. Michelle is always available to help—even at the shortest of notices. I am so grateful for her friendship and her belief in my ideas. Ben has been a delight to work with. He has been extraordinarily patient with my frequent delays, constructive in his criticism, and very careful in his reading of the manuscript. Every chapter of the manuscript benefited from Ben's sharp intellect, breadth of understanding, and editorial skills. Toward the end of the copyediting process, Gia Gonzales and Maury Botton showed incredible patience as I was often behind in meeting deadlines.

My family has always been there for me. My brother, Qasim, and his family; my sisters, Rabia and Fakiha, and their families; and my in-laws have always been a source of encouragement and support. I am grateful for their love every day.

A large portion of the book was written during the COVID-19 lockdowns. Those were difficult days, full of anxiety. Yet, I recognize that I was luckier than most. I was surrounded by love, light, and optimism. My wife, Afreen, and our children, Rahem and Samah, are the reason there is never any shortage of light in my life or joy in my heart. This book is dedicated to the warmth of their love and their infectious optimism for a better world.

Notes

PROLOGUE

1   Names have been changed for privacy.

2   Title 42 of the U.S. Code deals with public health, social welfare, and civil rights. It was passed in 1944 and was used by the Trump administration during the COVID-19 pandemic to turn away migrants and was kept in place by the Biden administration until May 2023. For more details on the history of the act, see chapter 9.

3   Robert Wilkins, "Under Pretext of Pandemic, Babies Born in US—Legal American Citizens—Expelled with Mothers to Mexico," *Common Dreams*, February 5, 2021, www.commondreams.org/news/2021/02/05/under-pretext-pandemic-babies-born-us-legal-american-citizens-expelled-mothers.

4   Tanvi Misra, "Revealed: US Citizen Newborns Sent to Mexico Under Trump-Era Border Ban," *The Guardian*, February 5, 2021.

5   While the ideas that built the foundations of germ theory were developed over decades, it was in the later part of the nineteenth century that the rapid progress in medicine and microbiology occurred that codified those ideas into postulates and theories that are now broadly called *germ theory*.

6   The issue of race and disease is well studied. Some resources with a particular focus on the United States can be accessed at "Racism and Health: A Reading List," Association of American Medical Colleges, www.aamc.org/news/racism-and-health-reading-list.

7   Cancer outcomes for historically marginalized communities in the United States are discussed in a number of studies. See, for example, Alicia L. Best et al., "Structural Racism and Cancer: Calls to Action for Cancer Researchers to Address Racial/Ethnic Cancer Inequity in the United States," *Cancer Epidemiology, Biomarkers and Prevention* 31, no. 6 (2022): 1243–46; Anna Stubblefield, "The Entanglement of Race and Cognitive Dis/Ability," *Metaphilosophy* 40, no. 3–4 (2009): 531–51; see, for example, Dorothy

Roberts, *Killing the Black Body: Race, Reproduction, and the Meaning of Liberty* (New York: Vintage Books, 2014). Also see Brittany D. Chambers et al., "Clinicians' Perspectives on Racism and Black Women's Maternal Health," *Women's Health Reports* 3, no. 1 (2022): 476–82. For underfunding in Indian Health Services, see Donald Warne and Linda Bane Frizzell, "American Indian Health Policy: Historical Trends and Contemporary Issues," *American Journal of Public Health* 104, no. S3 (2014): S263–67; Lia Maria Fulgaro, "Death by Apathy: Tolerance of the Government's Failure to Fund Promised Healthcare Causes Loss of Native American Lives," *Seattle Journal for Social Justice* 20, no. 2 (2021): 583.

1. THE CAMPAIGNS

1 The speech by President Obama is available at obamawhitehouse .archives.gov/blog/2011/05/02/osama-bin-laden-dead. For the news in Pakistan, see stories in the *Express Tribune*, tribune.com.pk/story/160514 /osama-bin-laden-killed-live-updates, and at *Dawn*, https://www.dawn .com/news/625466/osama-bin-laden-killed-in-pakistan-says-obama.

2 Associated Press, "US-Pakistan Relations 'at Turning Point' After Killing of Bin Laden, Warns Clinton," *The Guardian*, May 27, 2011. See also Declan Walsh, "Leaked Report Cites Pakistan's Failings Before U.S. Killed Bin Laden," *New York Times*, July 8, 2013.

3 Sara Reardon, "CIA's Fake Vaccination Drive Angers Public Health World," *Science*, July 13, 2011.

4 There are numerous news articles on Dr. Afridi and his interactions with the CIA. For details on some of them, see Umer Rahman, "Identity, Nationalism and Ethnic Divide: A Case Study on Dr. Shakil Afridi's Reputation," Florida International University Digital Commons, Asian Studies Theses, 2013, digitalcommons.fiu.edu/cgi/viewcontent.cgi ?article=1000&context=asianstudies_grad.

5 Saeed Shah, "CIA Organised Fake Vaccination Drive to Get Osama Bin Laden's Family DNA," *The Guardian*, July 11, 2011.

6 See the WHO's report on hepatitis in Pakistan, www.emro.who.int/pak /programmes/prevention-a-control-of-hepatitis.html.

7 World Health Organization, "15 Million People Affected with Hepatitis B and C in Pakistan: Government Announces Ambitious Plan to Eliminate Hepatitis," July 28, 2019, www.who.int/news/item/28-07-2019-15 -million-people-affected-with-hepatitis-b-and-c-in-pakistan-government -announces-ambitious-plan-to-eliminate-hepatitis.

8 Mishal S. Khan et al., "How Do External Donors Influence National Health Policy Processes? Experiences of Domestic Policy Actors in Cambodia and Pakistan," *Health Policy and Planning* 33, no. 2 (2018): 215–23.

9   Alexander Mullaney and Syeda Amna Hassan, "He Led the CIA to bin Laden—and Unwittingly Fueled a Vaccine Backlash," *National Geographic,* February 27, 2015, www.nationalgeographic.com/science/article/150227 -polio-pakistan-vaccination-taliban-osama-bin-laden.

10 Monica Martinez-Bravo and Andreas Stegmann, "In Vaccines We Trust? The Effects of the CIA's Vaccine Ruse on Immunization in Pakistan," *Journal of the European Economic Association* 20, no. 1 (2022): 150–86.

11 Saeed, "Fake Vaccination Drive." Also see Saeed Shah, "Health Workers Linked to CIA's Osama Bin Laden Assassination Plot Are Sacked," *The Guardian,* February 22, 2012.

12 See, for example, M. Ilyas Khan, "Pakistan's Army Ridiculed After Bin Laden Raid," *BBC News,* May 6, 2011; Julie McCarthy, "Pakistan Angry Over What It Didn't Know," *NPR Weekend Edition,* May 8, 2011.

13 See "66% of Pakistanis Don't Believe Osama bin Laden Was Killed: Poll," *Express Tribune,* May 6, 2011, tribune.com.pk/story/163178/66-of -pakistanis-dont-believe-osama-bin-laden-is-dead-poll.

14 Martinez-Bravo and Stegmann, "In Vaccines We Trust?"

15 The interview is available at www.cbsnews.com/news/the-defense-secretary -leon-panetta.

16 Mark Mazzetti, "Panetta Credits Pakistani Doctor in Bin Laden Raid," *New York Times,* January 28, 2012.

17 Ghulam Safdar, Abdul Wajid Khan, and Atif Ashraf, "Image of War on Terrorism into the Minds of Pakistani People," *The Government: Research Journal of Political Science* 6 (2017): 81–94.

18 Patrick B. Johnston and Anoop K. Sarbahi, "The Impact of US Drone Strikes on Terrorism in Pakistan," *International Studies Quarterly* 60, no. 2 (June 2016): 203–19.

19 Chris Woods, "Drones Causing Mass Trauma Among Civilians, Major Study Finds," *Bureau of Investigative Journalism,* September 25, 2012, www.thebureauinvestigates.com/stories/2012-09-25/drones-causing -mass-trauma-among-civilians-major-study-finds.

20 "Polio Eradication: The CIA and Their Unintended Victims," *The Lancet,* 383, no. 9932 (May 31, 2014): 1862.

21 Donald McNeil. "C.I.A. Vaccine Ruse May Have Harmed the War on Polio," *New York Times,* July 9, 2012.

22 Shazia Ghafoor and Nadeem Sheikh, "Eradication and Current Status of Poliomyelitis in Pakistan: Ground Realities," *Journal of Immunology Research* 2016, no. 1 (2016): 6837824.

23 José E. Hagan, "Progress Toward Polio Eradication: Worldwide, 2014– 2015," *CDC Morbidity and Mortality Weekly Report* 64, no. 19 (May 22, 2015): 527–31, www.cdc.gov/mmwr/preview/mmwrhtml/mm6419a5.htm #:~:text=During%202014%2C%20total%20of%20359,Horn%20of%20 Africa%20(Somalia%20and.

24   Jason Beaubien, "Taliban in Pakistan Derail World Polio Eradication," *NPR Morning Edition*, July 28, 2014, https://www.npr.org/sections/goatsand soda/2014/07/28/330767266/taliban-in-pakistan-derails-world-polio -eradication.
25   "Paying Polio Workers," *Express Tribune*, October 5, 2015, tribune.com.pk /story/967748/paying-polio-workers.
26   "Pakistan Suspends Polio Vaccination Campaign After Team Shot Dead," *Financial Times*, January 21, 2014, www.ft.com/content/2a6124ea-8299 -11e3-8119-00144feab7de.
27   Beaubien, "Taliban in Pakistan Derail World Polio Eradication."
28   Jon Boone, "Pakistan Shuts Down Save the Children Offices in Islamabad," *The Guardian*, June 12, 2015.
29   Muhammad H. Zaman, *We Wait for a Miracle: Health Care and the Forcibly Displaced* (Baltimore: Johns Hopkins University Press, 2023).
30   Gabriel E. Andrade and Azhar Hussain, "Polio in Pakistan: Political, Sociological, and Epidemiological Factors," *Cureus* 10, no. 10 (2018).
31   Meher Ahmed, "Pakistan Is Racing to Combat the World's First Extensively Drug-Resistant Typhoid Outbreak," *Scientific American*, March 14, 2018.
32   Qasim Mehmood et al., "COVID-19 Vaccine Hesitancy: Pakistan Struggles to Vaccinate Its Way Out of the Pandemic," *Therapeutic Advances in Vaccines and Immunotherapy* 10 (2022): 25151355221077658.
33   Karina Shah, "CIA's Hunt for Osama bin Laden Fueled Vaccine Hesitancy in Pakistan," *New Scientist*, May 11, 2021, www.newscientist.com /article/2277145-cias-hunt-for-osama-bin-laden-fuelled-vaccine-hesitancy -in-pakistan.
34   The program with Dr. Sultan is available at www.geo.tv/shows/aik-din -geo-ke-saath/353805-aik-din-geo-ke-sath-dr-faisal-sultan-06th-june -2021.
35   Jeanne Lenzer, "Fake Vaccine Campaign in Pakistan Could Threaten Plans to Eradicate Polio," *BMJ*, July 19, 2011, www.bmj.com/content/343 /bmj.d4580.full.
36   Donald G. McNeil, "Deans Condemn Vaccine Ruse Used in Bin Laden Hunt," *New York Times*, January 7, 2013.
37   Mark Mazzetti, "U.S. Cites End to C.I.A. Ruses Using Vaccines," *New York Times*, May 20, 2014.
38   Chris Bing and Joel Schectman, "Pentagon Ran Secret Anti-Vax Campaign to Undermine China During Pandemic," Reuters, June 14, 2024.
39   Victoria Milko, "Concern Among Muslims over Halal Status of COVID-19 Vaccine," *PBS News*, December 20, 2020.
40   Richard C. Paddock, "Is the Vaccine Halal? Indonesians Await the Answer," *New York Times*, January 5, 2021.
41   Bing and Schectman, "Pentagon Ran Secret Anti-Vax Campaign."

2. THE EXCEPTIONALISM OF INFECTION

1   Movies focused on infection found a renewed interest during the CO-VID-19 pandemic. For example, see *Exploring the Parallels Between Reality and Film: Outbreak, Contagion and the COVID-19 Pandemic*, National Emerging Special Pathogens Training and Education Center, July 31, 2023, netec.org/2023/07/31/exploring-the-parallels-between-reality-and-film-outbreak-contagion-the-covid-19-pandemic.

2   John Dugdale, "Plague Fiction: Why Authors Love to Write About Pandemics," *The Guardian*, August 1, 2014. See also Jeffrey S. Sartin, "Contagious Horror: Infectious Themes in Fiction and Film," *Clinical Medicine and Research* 17, no. 1–2 (2019): 41–46, doi:10.3121/cmr.2019.1432.

3   Donatella Lippi, Elena Varotto, Simon Donell, and Francesco M. Galassi, "Dino Buzzati's 50th Death Anniversary: An Appraisal of Medicine and Infectivology's Influence on His Literary Production," *Acta Bio Medica: Atenei Parmensis* 93, no. 5 (2022).

4   https://archive.org/details/michaeldolstr.ibnalwardiontheplague1974/mode/2up

5   B. Bastian et al., "Explaining Illness with Evil: Pathogen Prevalence Fosters Moral Vitalism," *Proceedings of the Royal Society B* 286 (1914): 20191576.

6   Hans Zinsser, *Rats, Lice and History* (Boston: Little, Brown, 1935).

7   R.I. Duffus, "Man's War Against Pestilence: Dr. Zinsser Makes a Remarkable Excursion into History," *New York Times*, February 17, 1935, www.nytimes.com/1935/02/17/archives/mans-war-against-pestilence-dr-zinsser-makes-a-remarkable-excursion.html; J. Howard Mueller, "Hans Zinsser 1878–1940," *Journal of Bacteriology* 40, no. 6 (1940): i2–753. Also see Zinsser's autobiography *As I Remember Him: Biography of R.S.* (Boston: Little, Brown, 1940).

8   Larry Lutwick, "Brill-Zinsser Disease," *The Lancet* 357, no. 9263 (2001): 1198–1200.

9   P.M. Dunn, "Oliver Wendell Holmes (1809–1894) and His Essay on Puerperal Fever," *ADC Fetal and Neonatal* 92, no. 4 (2007): F325, doi: 10.1136/adc.2005.077578; Nawal El Saadawi, *The Essential Nawal El Saadawi: A Reader* (London: Bloomsbury, 2010).

10 Several biographies of Chekhov talk about his overlapping interests and how his writing was influenced by his medical training: Anton Chekhov, *Ward No. 6 and Other Stories, 1892–1895* (New York: Penguin, 2002); Jack Coulehan, ed., *Chekhov's Doctors: A Collection of Chekhov's Medical Tales* (Kent, OH: Kent State University Press, 2003). Also see Alexander Macdonald, "Anton Chekhov: The Physician and Major Writer," *JAMA* 229, no. 9 (1974): 1203–4; Jon Lellenberg, Daniel Stashower, and Charles Foley, eds., *Arthur Conan Doyle: A Life in Letters* (London: Penguin, 2008).

11 See, for example, Joshua Lederberg, "Infectious History," *Science* 288, no. 5464 (2000): 287–93; Macfarlane Burnet and David O. White, *Natural*

History of Infectious Disease (Cambridge: Cambridge University Press, 1972); P.W. Ewald, *Evolution of Infectious Disease* (New York: Oxford University Press, 1994).

12   See Martha R.J. Clokie, Andrew D. Millard, Andrey V. Letarov, and Shaun Heaphy, "Phages in Nature," *Bacteriophage* 1, no. 1 (2011): 31–45; R. Calendar, ed., *The Bacteriophages*, Vol. 2 (New York: Oxford University Press, 2006).

13   There is vast literature on the history of epidemics and pandemics and how they shaped human history. See, for example, Sheldon J. Watts, *Epidemics and History: Disease, Power, and Imperialism* (New Haven, CT: Yale University Press, 1999); Jo N. Hays, *Epidemics and Pandemics: Their Impacts on Human History* (New York: Bloomsbury, 2005); Jocelyne Piret and Guy Boivin, "Pandemics Throughout History," *Frontiers in Microbiology* 11 (2021): 631736; Mitchell L. Hammond, *Epidemics and the Modern World* (Toronto: University of Toronto Press, 2020).

14   See Christer Bruun, "The Antonine Plague and the 'Third-Century Crisis,'" in *Crises and the Roman Empire*, ed. Olivier Hekster, Gerda de Kleijn, and Daniëlle Slootjes (Leiden: Brill, 2007), 201–17; Richard P. Duncan-Jones, "The Impact of the Antonine Plague," *Journal of Roman Archaeology*, no. 9 (1996): 108–36.

15   Jennifer Manley, "Measles and Ancient Plagues: A Note on New Scientific Evidence," *Classical World* 107, no. 3 (2014): 393–97.

16   William Rosen, *Justinian's Flea: The First Great Plague and the End of the Roman Empire* (London: Penguin, 2007); Peter Sarris, "Viewpoint New Approaches to the 'Plague of Justinian,'" *Past and Present* 254, no. 1 (2022): 315–46; Peter Sarris, "The Justinianic Plague: Origins and Effects," *Continuity and Change* 17, no. 2 (2002): 169–82.

17   Lester K. Little, ed., *Plague and the End of Antiquity: The Pandemic of 541–750* (Cambridge: Cambridge University Press, 2007).

18   There is vast literature on the Black Death, its origin, and its impact. See, for example, the following books and references within: Robert S. Gottfried, *Black Death* (New York: Simon and Schuster, 2010); Norman F. Cantor, *In the Wake of the Plague: The Black Death and the World It Made* (New York: Simon and Schuster, 2014); Ole J. Benedictow, *The Black Death, 1346–1353: The Complete History* (Martlesham, UK: Boydell Press, 2004).

19   Rodolfo Acuña-Soto et al., "Drought, Epidemic Disease, and the Fall of Classic Period Cultures in Mesoamerica (AD 750–950). Hemorrhagic Fevers as a Cause of Massive Population Loss," *Medical Hypotheses* 65, no. 2 (2005).

20   Rodolfo Acuña-Soto, Leticia Calderón Romero, and James H. Maguire, "Large Epidemics of Hemorrhagic Fevers in Mexico 1545–1815," *American Journal of Tropical Medicine and Hygiene* 62, no. 6 (2000): 733–39.

21   For hate, blame, and scapegoating, see Samuel K. Cohn, "Pandemics: Waves of Disease, Waves of Hate from the Plague of Athens to AIDS," *Historical Research* 85, no. 230 (2012): 535–55.

22   Samuel K. Cohn Jr., "The Black Death and the Burning of Jews," *Past and Present* 196, no. 1 (2007): 3–36.

23   Albert Winkler, "The Medieval Holocaust: The Approach of the Plague and the Destruction of Jews in Germany, 1348–1349," BYU Faculty Publications, 2005, scholarsarchive.byu.edu/cgi/viewcontent.cgi?article=2841&context=facpub.

24   Paul Weindling, *Epidemics and Genocide in Eastern Europe, 1890–1945* (Oxford: Oxford University Press, 2000).

25   Joseph L. Miller, "History of Syphilis," *Annals of Medical History* 2, no. 4 (1930): 394.

26   Ernest Lawrence Abel, "Syphilis: The History of an Eponym," *Names* 66, no. 2 (2018): 96–102.

27   Katarzyna Plagens-Rotman et al., "Syphilis: Then and Now," *Advances in Dermatology and Allergology/Postępy Dermatologii i Alergologii* 38, no. 4 (2021): 550–54.

28   Antonio Tagarelli, Giuseppe Tagarelli, Paolo Lagonia, and Anna Piro, "Morbus Europaeus: Europeans Naming Syphilis for Their Enemies," *Archives of Dermatology* 148, no. 7 (2012): 831–31.

29   Mircea Tampa et al., "Brief History of Syphilis," *Journal of Medicine and Life* 7, no. 1 (2014): 4.

30   Justus Friedrich Carl Hecker, *The Epidemics of the Middle Ages* (Philadelphia: Haswell, Barrington, and Haswell, 1838).

31   Miasma has been a topic of great interest among historians, epidemiologists, and other public health researchers. For a good introduction, see Carlo M. Cipolla, *Miasmas and Disease: Public Health and the Environment in the Pre-Industrial Age* (New Haven, CT: Yale University Press, 1992).

32   Ajesh Kannadan, "History of the Miasma Theory of Disease," *Essai* 16, no. 1 (2018): 18.

33   Sylvia N. Tesh, "Miasma and 'Social Factors' in Disease Causality: Lessons from the Nineteenth Century," *Journal of Health Politics, Policy and Law* 20, no. 4 (1995): 1001–24.

34   For an accessible account of Snow's work, see Steven Johnson, *The Ghost Map: The Story of London's Most Terrifying Epidemic—and How It Changed Science, Cities, and the Modern World* (New York: Penguin, 2006).

35   Donald Cameron and Ian G. Jones, "John Snow, the Broad Street Pump and Modern Epidemiology," *International Journal of Epidemiology* 12, no. 4 (1983): 393–96.

36   Alexander Kappes et al., "Livestock Health and Disease Economics: A Scoping Review of Selected Literature," *Frontiers in Veterinary Science*, no. 10 (2023): 1168649.

37   B. Bett, "Effects of Climate Change on the Occurrence and Distribution of Livestock Diseases," *Preventive Veterinary Medicine*, no. 137 (2017): 119–29.

38 Mullusew Gashaw, "A Review on Avian Influenza and Its Economic and Public Health Impact," *International Journal of Veterinary Science and Technology* 4, no. 1 (2020): 15–27.

39 Ramadan Abdelmoez Farahat, Sheharyar Hassan Khan, Ali A. Rabaan, and Jaffar A. Al-Tawfiq, "The Resurgence of Avian Influenza and Human Infection: A Brief Outlook," *New Microbes and New Infections*, no. 53 (2023).

40 For an accessible overview of zoonotic diseases, see David Quammen, *Spillover: Animal Infections and the Next Human Pandemic* (New York: W.W. Norton, 2012). Also see World Health Organization, "A Brief Guide to Emerging Infectious Diseases and Zoonoses," 2014, iris.who.int/handle/10665/204722.

41 George M. Baer, ed., *The Natural History of Rabies* (New York: Routledge, 2017). Also see James H. Steele and Peter J. Fernandez, "History of Rabies and Global Aspects," in *The Natural History of Rabies*, ed. George M. Baer (New York: Routledge, 2017), 1–24.

42 D.J. Hicks, A.R. Fooks, and N. Johnson, "Developments in Rabies Vaccines," *Clinical and Experimental Immunology* 169, no. 3 (2012): 199–204.

43 For an overview of research on plague, see Kenneth L. Gage and Michael Y. Kosoy, "Natural History of Plague: Perspectives from More Than a Century of Research," *Annual Review of Entomology* 50, no. 1 (2005): 505–28. For a description of the biological aspects of the disease, see Susan Scott and Christopher J. Duncan, *Biology of Plagues: Evidence from Historical Populations* (Cambridge: Cambridge University Press, 2001).

44 Vladimir V. Nikiforov, He Gao, Lei Zhou, and Andrey Anisimov, "Plague: Clinics, Diagnosis and Treatment," in *Yersinia pestis: Retrospective and Perspective*, ed. Ruifu Yang and Andrey Anisimov (New York: Springer, 2016), 293–312.

45 Thomas Butler, "Plague into the 21st Century," *Clinical Infectious Diseases* 49, no. 5 (2009): 736–42; Leslie A. Reperant and Albert DME Osterhaus, "AIDS, Avian Flu, SARS, MERS, Ebola, Zika…What Next?," *Vaccine* 35, no. 35 (2017): 4470–74.

46 There is ongoing debate on whether COVID-19 was a zoonotic disease or a gain of function experiment that went wrong. For details on the controversy see Lawrence O. Gostin and Gigi K. Gronvall, "The Origins of Covid-19—Why It Matters (and Why It Doesn't)," *New England Journal of Medicine* 388, no. 25 (2023): 2305–8 and the House Oversight Committee Report from 2023, https://oversight.house.gov/release/final-report-covid-select-concludes-2-year-investigation-issues-500-page-final-report-on-lessons-learned-and-the-path-forward.

47 Abroo Aman Andrabi, "Islamic Perspective of Plagues and Pandemics," *International Journal of Humanities, Social Sciences and Education*, no. 9 (2022): 41–50.

48 Gian Franco Gensini, Magdi H. Yacoub, and Andrea A. Conti, "The Concept of Quarantine in History: From Plague to SARS," *Journal of Infection* 49, no. 4 (2004): 257–61.

49 For a short visual description of quarantine over time, see Peter Tyson, "A Short History of Quarantine," *Nova*, PBS, October 12, 2004, www.pbs.org /wgbh/nova/article/short-history-of-quarantine.

50 Eugenia Tognotti. "Lessons from the History of Quarantine, from Plague to Influenza A," *Emerging Infectious Diseases Journal* 19, no. 2 (February 2013), wwwnc.cdc.gov/eid/article/19/2/12-0312_article.

51 Ibid.

52 For an overview of the development of germ theory, see Robert P. Gaynes, *Germ Theory: Medical Pioneers in Infectious Diseases* (New York: Wiley, 2023); Richard Harrison Shryock, "Germ Theories in Medicine Prior to 1870: Further Comments on Continuity in Science," in *Clio Medica. Acta Academiae Internationalis Historiae Medicinae*, vol. 7, pp. 81–109 (Brill, 1972), doi.org/10.1163/9789004418196_006; James Trostle, "Early Work in Anthropology and Epidemiology: From Social Medicine to the Germ Theory, 1840 to 1920," in *Anthropology and Epidemiology: Interdisciplinary Approaches to the Study of Health and Disease*, ed. Craig R. Janes (Dordrecht: Springer, 1986), 35–57.

53 For an accessible account of the developments in microbiology in Europe in the late nineteenth century, see William Rosen, *Miracle Cure: The Creation of Antibiotics and the Birth of Modern Medicine* (New York: Penguin, 2017).

54 Koch and Pasteur have been studied extensively. See Gaynes, *Germ Theory,* for an accessible account. Also see Muhammad Hamid Zaman, *Biography of Resistance* (New York: HarperCollins, 2020); Agnes Ullmann, "Pasteur-Koch: Distinctive Ways of Thinking About Infectious Diseases," *Microbe-American Society for Microbiology* 2, no. 8 (2007): 383; John Waller, The Discovery of the Germ: Twenty Years That Transformed the Way We Think About Disease" (New York: Columbia University Press, 2002); J. Andrew Mendelsohn, "'Like All That Lives': Biology, Medicine and Bacteria in the Age of Pasteur and Koch," *History and Philosophy of the Life Sciences* 24, no. 1 (2002): 3–36.

55 Robert Koch, *Die Ätiologie der Milzbrand-Krankheit, begründet auf die Entwicklungsgeschichte des Bacillus Anthracis* (1876), Vol. 9 (Barth, 1910).

56 Gerald B. Webb, "Robert Koch [1843–1910]," *Annals of Medical History* 4, no. 6 (1932): 509.

57 For a discussion of Pasteur's life, work, impact, and legacy, see Patrice Debré, *Louis Pasteur* (Baltimore: Johns Hopkins University Press, 2000).

58 Stefan Riedel, "Edward Jenner and the History of Smallpox and Vaccination," *Baylor University Medical Center Proceedings* 18, no. 1 (2005): 21–25.

59 Peter C.B. Turnbull, "Anthrax Vaccines: Past, Present and Future," *Vaccine* 9, no. 8 (1991): 533–39.

60   Gaynes, *Germ Theory*.

61   Emmanuelle Cambau and Michael Drancourt, "Steps Towards the Discovery of Mycobacterium Tuberculosis by Robert Koch, 1882," *Clinical Microbiology and Infection* 20, no. 3 (2014): 196–201.

62   Mohammad Sirajul Islam, Bohumil S. Drasar, and R. Bradley Sack, "The Aquatic Environment as a Reservoir of Vibrio Cholerae: A Review," *Journal of Diarrhoeal Diseases Research* (1993): 197–206.

63   Robert Koch, "An Address on Cholera and Its Bacillus," *British Medical Journal* 2, no. 1236 (1884): 453.

64   Attila Horváth, "Biology and Natural History of Syphilis," in *Sexually Transmitted Infections and Sexually Transmitted Diseases*, ed. Gerd Gross and Stephen K. Tyring (Berlin: Springer, 2011), 129–41.

65   For a detailed discussion of the Tuskegee study, see Susan M. Reverby, ed., *Tuskegee's Truths: Rethinking the Tuskegee Syphilis Study* (Chapel Hill: University of North Carolina Press, 2012). Also chapter 6 in this book.

66   Hubert Lechevalier, "Dmitri Iosifovich Ivanovski (1864–1920)," *Bacteriological Reviews* 36, no. 2 (1972): 135–45.

67   L. Bos, "Beijerinck's Work on Tobacco Mosaic Virus: Historical Context and Legacy," Philosophical Transactions of the Royal Society of London, Series B, *Biological Sciences* 354, no. 1383 (1999): 675–85.

68   Gulten Dinc and Yesim Isil Ulman, "The Introduction of Variolation 'A La Turca' to the West by Lady Mary Montagu and Turkey's Contribution to This," *Vaccine* 25, no. 21 (2007): 4261–65.

69   Among the several biographies of Jenner is a detailed two-volume biography that covers his life, work, and legacy: John Baron, *The Life of Edward Jenner MD* (Cambridge: Cambridge University Press, 2014).

70   Paul E.M. Fine, "Herd Immunity: History, Theory, Practice," *Epidemiologic Reviews* 15, no. 2 (1993): 265–302.

71   Gian Franco Gensini, Andrea Alberto Conti, and Donatella Lippi, "The Contributions of Paul Ehrlich to Infectious Disease," *Journal of Infection* 54, no. 3 (2007): 221–24. Also see Florian Winau, Otto Westphal, and Rolf Winau, "Paul Ehrlich: In Search of the Magic Bullet," *Microbes and Infection* 6, no. 8 (2004): 786–89.

72   William Rosen, *Miracle Cure: The Creation of Antibiotics and the Birth of Modern Medicine* (New York: Penguin, 2017).

73   For a discussion of evolution and politics of phage therapy, see Nina Chanishvili, "Phage Therapy: History from Twort and d'Herelle Through Soviet Experience to Current Approaches," *Advances in Virus Research*, no. 83 (2012): 3–40; William C. Summers, "The Strange History of Phage Therapy," *Bacteriophage* 2, no. 2 (2012): 130–33; Zaman, *Biography of Resistance*.

74   William C. Summers, "On the Origins of the Science in Arrowsmith: Paul de Kruif, Felix d'Herelle, and Phage," *Journal of the History of Medicine and Allied Sciences* 46, no. 3 (1991): 315–32.

75 William C. Summers, "The Cold War and Phage Therapy: How Geo-
politics Stalled Development of Viruses as Antibacterials," *Annual Review of Virology*, no. 11 (2024).

76 Zaman, *Biography of Resistance.*

77 Matthew R. Smallman-Raynor and Andrew D. Cliff, "Impact of Infectious Diseases on War," *Infectious Disease Clinics* 18, no. 2 (2004): 341–68; Hugh Pennington, "The Impact of Infectious Disease in War Time: A Look Back at WWI," *Future Microbiology* 14, no. 3 (2019): 165–68; Roberto Biselli et al., "A Historical Review of Military Medical Strategies for Fighting Infectious Diseases: From Battlefields to Global Health," *Biomedicines* 10, no. 8 (2022): 2050.

78 For a comprehensive account of the discovery and production of penicillin, see Robert Bud, *Penicillin: Triumph and Tragedy* (Oxford: Oxford University Press, 2007).

79 Antimicrobial resistance is one of the most pressing global health issues of our time. For a general overview, see Julian Davies and Dorothy Davies, "Origins and Evolution of Antibiotic Resistance," *Microbiology and Molecular Biology Reviews* 74, no. 3 (2010): 417–33; Zaman, *Biography of Resistance*; R. Craig MacLean and Alvaro San Millan, "The Evolution of Antibiotic Resistance," *Science* 365, no. 6458 (2019): 1082–83 and references therein.

3. THE DISEASE AND THE OUTSIDER

1 Kimmy Yam, "Donald Trump Touts Racial Equality While Referring to COVID-19 as 'China Plague,'" *NBC News*, June 5, 2020.

2 For a detailed account of the history of race, politics, and the Chinese Exclusion Act, see Andrew Gyory, *Closing the Gate: Race, Politics, and the Chinese Exclusion Act* (Chapel Hill: University of North Carolina Press, 1998); Erika Lee, *At America's Gates: Chinese Immigration During the Exclusion Era, 1882–1943* (Chapel Hill: University of North Carolina Press, 2003).

3 Charles J. McClain, *In Search of Equality: The Chinese Struggle Against Discrimination in Nineteenth-Century America* (Berkeley: University of California Press, 1994).

4 Joan B. Trauner, "The Chinese as Medical Scapegoats in San Francisco, 1870–1905," *California History* 57, no. 1 (1978): 70–87.

5 Sucheng Chan, "Chinese Livelihood in Rural California: The Impact of Economic Change, 1860–1880," *Pacific Historical Review* 53, no. 3 (1984): 273–307.

6 Joseph Camp Griffith Kennedy, "Population of the United States in 1860: Compiled from the Original Returns of the Eighth Census, Under the Direction of the Secretary of the Interior," Vol. 1 (Washington, DC: GPO, 1990).

7   Burlingame-Seward Treaty, "Peace, Amity, and Commerce," US-China 16 (1868); Chinese-Americans 1785: Demographics, https://libguides.south ernct.edu/c.php?g=15048&p=81577. Also see Roger Daniels, *Asian America: Chinese and Japanese in the United States Since 1850* (Seattle: University of Washington Press, 2011).

8   Doyce B. Nunis, Denis Kearney, and J. Bryce, "The Demagogue and the Demographer: Correspondence of Denis Kearney and Lord Bryce," *Pacific Historical Review* 36, no. 3 (1967): 269–88.

9   Chew Heong v. United States, 112 U.S. 536 (1884), p. 566.

10 The PBS American Experience Series "The Chinese Exclusion Act" provides a visually captivating background on the issue, www.pbs.org/wgbh /americanexperience/films/chinese-exclusion-act.

11 For a detailed account of the history of race, politics, and the Chinese Exclusion Act, see Andrew Gyory, *Closing the Gate: Race, Politics, and the Chinese Exclusion Act* (Chapel Hill: University of North Carolina Press, 1998); Erika Lee, *At America's Gates: Chinese Immigration During the Exclusion Era, 1882–1943* (Chapel Hill: University of North Carolina Press, 2003)..

12 Bailey DeSimone, "The Chinese Exclusion Act, Part 2: The Legacy," Library of Congress Blogs, May 16, 2022, blogs.loc.gov/law/2022/05/the -chinese-exclusion-act-part-2-the-legacy/#:~:text=Though%20commen-tators%20across%20the%20country,grew%20by%20just%201%2C852 %20people.

13 Yen Tzu-Kuei, "Rock Springs Incident," *Chinese Studies in History* 7, no. 3 (1974): 51–66; R. Gregory Nokes, "'A Most Daring Outrage': Murders at Chinese Massacre Cove, 1887," *Oregon Historical Quarterly* 107, no. 3 (2006): 326–53.

14 Text of Geary Act available at loveman.sdsu.edu/docs/1892GearyAct .pdf.

15 Fong Yue Ting v. United States, 149 U.S. 698 (1893). Available at supreme .justia.com/cases/federal/us/149/698.

16 Trauner, "Chinese as Medical Scapegoats," 70–87.

17 For the images that connected disease, hygiene, and race, see Trauner, "Chinese as Medical Scapegoats," 70–87. Also see Michelle Bae-Dimitriadis, "Antiracist Visual Critique: Dis-ease (ing) of the Mythmaking of Asian Immigrants in Political Cartoons," *Art Education* 74, no. 6 (2021): 55–57; Yii-Jan Lin, "An Apocalyptic Epidemiology of Foreignness: The Use of Revelation in American Associations of Immigrants with Disease," *Divided Worlds? Challenges in Classics and New Testament Studies* 100 (2023): 83; Nayan Shah, *Contagious Divides: Epidemics and Race in San Francisco's Chinatown*, Vol. 7 (Berkeley: University of California Press, 2001).

18 Trauner, "Chinese as Medical Scapegoats," 70–87.

19 San Francisco Board of Supervisors, Municipal Reports (1876–1877) p. 394.

20   Arthur B. Stout, "Impurity Of Race, as a Cause of Decay," First Biennial Report of the State Board of Health of California for the Years 1870 and 1871 (D. W. Gelwicks, 1871), 7.

21   Report of Special Committee on the Condition of the Chinese Quarter" Municipal Reports, 1885, p. 208.

22   Leprosy has long been associated with racism. For background about the historical relationship, see Zachary Gussow and George S. Tracy, "Stigma and the Leprosy Phenomenon: The Social History of a Disease in the Nineteenth and Twentieth Centuries," *Bulletin of the History of Medicine* 44, no. 5 (1970): 425–49.

23   John R. Trautman, "A Brief History of Hansen's Disease," *Bulletin of the New York Academy of Medicine* 60, no. 7 (1984): 689.

24   "Examination of the Testimony of John L. Meares, MD, on Oct. 24, 1876 Before Joint Special Committee to Investigate Chinese Immigration," *Report of the Royal Commission on Chinese Immigration: Report and Evidence* (Ottawa: Order of the Royal Commission, 1885), 198.

25   Sana Loue, *Gender, Ethnicity, and Health Research* (New York: Kluwer Academic, 1999). Also discussed in Pam Fessler, "Before 'Kung Flu' There Was the Asian Shaming of Leprosy," *Daily Beast*, July 26, 2020.

26   Ibid.

27   Trauner, "Chinese as Medical Scapegoats," 70–87.

28   Hidetaka Hirota, "Immigration to American Cities, 1800–1924," in *Oxford Research Encyclopedia of American History*, November 20, 2018, oxfordre.com/americanhistory/view/10.1093/acrefore/9780199329175 .001.0001/acrefore-9780199329175-e-577.

29   Howard Markel and Alexandra Minna Stern, "The Foreignness of Germs: The Persistent Association of Immigrants and Disease in American Society," *Milbank Quarterly* 80, no. 4 (2002): 757–88.

30   John Higham, *Strangers in the Land: Patterns of American Nativism, 1860–1925* (New Brunswick, NJ: Rutgers University Press, 2002).

31   Ibid.

32   Howard Markel and Alexandra Minna Stern, "Which Face? Whose Nation? Immigration, Public Health, and the Construction of Disease at America's Ports and Borders, 1891–1928," *American Behavioral Scientist* 42, no. 9 (1999): 1314–31.

33   Howard Markel, "'The Eyes Have It': Trachoma, the Perception of Disease, the United States Public Health Service, and the American Jewish Immigration Experience, 1897–1924." *Bulletin of the History of Medicine* 74, no. 3 (2000): 525–60.

34   *U.S. Public Health Service (USPHS) Annual Reports of the Surgeon General of the USPHS* (Washington, DC: GPO, 1912–30).

35   Roger Daniels, "No Lamps Were Lit for Them: Angel Island and the Historiography of Asian American Immigration," *Journal of American Ethnic History* (1997): 3–18; Lucy E. Salyer, *Laws Harsh as Tigers: Chinese Im-*

migrants and the Shaping of Modern Immigration Law (Chapel Hill: University of North Carolina Press, 1995).

36 Howard Markel and Alexandra Minna Stern, "The Foreignness of Germs: The Persistent Association of Immigrants and Disease in American Society," *Milbank Quarterly* 80, no. 4 (2002): 757–88.

37 Ben Freedman, "The First State Board of Health Laboratories in the United States," *Public Health Reports* 69, no. 9 (1954): 867.

38 John F. Anderson, "Organization, Powers, and Duties of the United States Public Health Service Today," *American Journal of Public Health* 3, no. 9 (1913): 845–52.

39 Health and Human Services Department, "Control of Communicable Diseases; Foreign Quarantine: Suspension of the Right to Introduce and Prohibition of Introduction of Persons into United States from Designated Foreign Countries or Places for Public Health Purposes," September 11, 2020, 42 CFR Part 71 [Docket No. CDC-2020-0033], RIN 0920-AA76, www.federalregister.gov/d/2020-20036.

40 J.J. Kinyoun and W. Wyman "Plague in San Francisco" (1900), Public health reports (Washington, DC, 1974), 121 Suppl 1, 17–16.

41 Ryan M. Alexander, "The Fever of War: Epidemic Typhus and Public Health in Revolutionary Mexico City, 1915–1917," *Hispanic American Historical Review* 100, no. 1 (2020): 63–92.

42 Claude Pierce, "Combating Typhus Fever on the Mexican Border," *Public Health Reports (1896–1970)* 32, no. 12 (March 23, 1917).

43 H. Markel and A. M. Stern, "The Foreignness of Germs: The Persistent Association of Immigrants and Disease in American Society," *Milbank Quarterly* 80, no. 4 (2002): 757–88, v. doi: 10.1111/1468-0009.00030.

44 Ibid.

45 See https://www.tallahassee.com/story/news/local/state/2021/08/12/are-migrants-bringing-covid-19-to-florida/8101828002/ and https://www.the guardian.com/world/2021/aug/12/covid-19-texas-migrants-facts.

46 For detailed results, see the American Presidency Project, www.presidency.ucsb.edu/statistics/elections/1928.

47 A.W. Hedrich, "The Movements of Epidemic Meningitis, 1915–1930," *Public Health Reports (1896–1970)* (1931): 2709–26.

48 J.C. Perry, "Incidence and Source of Epidemic Meningitis on the Pacific Coast 1929," *American Journal of Public Health and the Nations Health* 21, no. 2 (1931): 171–76.

49 Executive Order 5143—Restricting for the Time Being the Transportation of Passengers from Certain Ports in the Orient to a United States Port, June 21, 1929, www.presidency.ucsb.edu/documents/executive-order-5143-restricting-for-the-time-being-the-transportation-passengers-from.

50 Library of Congress, "Immigration and Relocation in U.S. History," www.loc.gov/classroom-materials/immigration/chinese/growth-and-inclusion

/#:~:text=Despite%20continuing%20restrictions%20in%20immigra
tion,the%20mainstream%20of%20U.S.%20society.

51 Mae M. Ngai, "The Architecture of Race in American Immigration Law: An Examination of the Immigration Act of 1924," in *Race, Law and Society* (London: Routledge, 2017), 351–76.

52 Library of Congress, "Immigration and Relocation."

53 Executive Order 5143 by President Hoover, June 21, 1929, https://www.presidency.ucsb.edu/documents/executive-order-5143-restricting-for-the-time-being-the-transportation-passengers-from.

54 Executive Order 5143—Restricting for the Time Being the Transportation of Passengers from Certain Ports in the Orient to a United States Port, June 21, 1929, www.presidency.ucsb.edu/documents/executive-order-5143-restricting-for-the-time-being-the-transportation-passengers-from.

55 J.C. Perry, "Incidence and Source of Epidemic Meningitis on the Pacific Coast 1929."

56 Ibid.

57 J.C. Geiger, "Control Measures Adopted for Epidemic Cerebrospinal Fever on Ships," *American Journal of Public Health and the Nations Health* 21, no. 2 (1931): 163–70.

58 Perry, "Incidence and Source."

59 Perry, "Incidence and Source."

4. IMPORTING AND EXPORTING CHOLERA

1 Richard A. Finkelstein, "Cholera, Vibrio cholerae O1 and O139, and Other Pathogenic Vibrios," in *Medical Microbiology*, 4th ed. (Galveston: University of Texas Medical Branch, 1996).

2 M.N. Guentzel and L.J. Berry, "Motility as a Virulence Factor for *Vibrio cholerae*," *Infection and Immunity* 11, no. 5 (1975): 890–97.

3 Mark Harrison, "A Dreadful Scourge: Cholera in Early Nineteenth-Century India," *Modern Asian Studies* 54, no. 2 (2020): 502–53.

4 Eric J. Nelson et al., "Cholera Transmission: The Host, Pathogen and Bacteriophage Dynamic," *Nature Reviews Microbiology* 7, no. 10 (2009): 693–702.

5 "Cholera," Mayo Clinic, www.mayoclinic.org/diseases-conditions/cholera/symptoms-causes/syc-20355287#.

6 Alexandra E. Purdy and Paula I. Watnick, "Spatially Selective Colonization of the Arthropod Intestine Through Activation of *Vibrio cholerae* Biofilm Formation," *Proceedings of the National Academy of Sciences* 108, no. 49 (2011): 19737–42.

7 Dawn L. Taylor, Tanya M. Kahawita, Sandy Cairncross, and Jeroen HJ Ensink, "The Impact of Water, Sanitation and Hygiene Interventions to Control Cholera: A Systematic Review," *PLOS One* 10, no. 8 (2015): e0135676.

8   Several studies talk about Pacini's work. For example, see D. Lippi, E. Gotuzzo, and S. Caini, "Cholera," *Microbiol Spectrum* 4, no. 4 (2016): PoH-0012-2015, doi:10.1128/microbiolspec.poH-0012-2015; Marina Bentivoglio and Paolo Pacini, "Filippo Pacini: A Determined Observer," *Brain Research Bulletin* 38, no. 2 (1995): 161–65; Donatella Lippi and Eduardo Gotuzzo, "The Greatest Steps Towards the Discovery of *Vibrio cholerae*," *Clinical Microbiology and Infection* 20, no. 3 (2014): 191–95.

9   John Snow, *On the Mode of Communication of Cholera* (London: John Churchill, 1855).

10   Donald Cameron and Ian G. Jones, "John Snow, the Broad Street Pump and Modern Epidemiology," *International Journal of Epidemiology* 12, no. 4 (1983): 393–96.

11   Several studies talk about Pacini's work. For example, see D. Lippi, E. Gotuzzo, and S. Caini, *Microbiology Spectrum* 4, no.10 (2016):1128, micro-biolspec.poh-0012-2015; Marina Bentivoglio and Paolo Pacini, "Filippo Pacini: A Determined Observer," *Brain Research Bulletin* 38, no. 2 (1995):161–65; Donatella Lippi and Eduardo Gotuzzo, "The Greatest Steps Towards the Discovery of Vibrio cholerae," *Clinical Microbiology and Infection* 20, no. 3 (2014): 191-95. Also see Aria Shakeri, "Filippo Pacini—A Life of Achievement," *JAMA Dermatology* 154, no. 3 (2018): 300; Claudio Pogliano, "Eye, Mind, Hand: Filippo Pacini's Microscopy," *Nuncius* 28, no. 2 (2013): 313–44.

12   Lippi, Gotuzzo, and Caini, "Cholera."

13   Edgar Erskine Hume, *Max Von Pettenkofer, His Theory of the Etiology of Cholera, Typhoid Fever and Other Intestinal Diseases: A Review of His Arguments and Evidence* (New York: P.B. Hoeber, 1927). Also see Alfredo Morabia, "Epidemiologic Interactions, Complexity, and the Lonesome Death of Max von Pettenkofer," *American Journal of Epidemiology* 166, no. 11 (2007): 1233–38.

14   Julia C. van Kessel and Andrew Camilli, "*Vibrio cholerae*: A Fundamental Model System for Bacterial Genetics and Pathogenesis Research," *Journal of Bacteriology* (2024): e00248-24.

15   Norman Howard-Jones, "Robert Koch and the *Cholera vibrio*: A Centenary," *British Medical Journal* (Clinical research ed.) 288, no. 6414 (1984): 379.

16   Lippi and Gotuzzo, "Greatest Steps."

17   Sambhu Nath De, *Cholera: Its Pathology and Pathogenesis* (Edinburgh: Oliver and Boyd, 1961).

18   Ciara Boylan, "Famine," in *The Princeton History of Modern Ireland*, ed. Richard Bourke and Ian McBride (Princeton, NJ: Princeton University Press, 2016), 409, citing James S. Donnelly Jr., *The Great Irish Potato Famine* (Thrupp, Stroud: Sutton Publishing, 2001), 181.

19   Several books have discussed the issue of disease as well as perceptions about the Irish in the United States. See for example Meredith B. Linn,

From Typhus to Tuberculosis and Fractures in Between: A Visceral Historical Archaeology of Irish Immigrant Life in New York City 1845–1870 (New York: Columbia University, 2008); Meredith B. Linn, *Irish Fever: An Archaeology of Illness, Injury, and Healing in New York City, 1845–1875* (Knoxville: University of Tennessee Press, 2024).

20   Walter J. Daly, "The Black Cholera Comes to the Central Valley of America in the 19th Century—1832, 1849, and Later," *Transactions of the American Clinical and Climatological Association*, no. 119 (2008): 143.

21   Library of Congress, "Adaptation and Assimilation," www.loc.gov /classroom-materials/immigration/irish/adaptation-and-assimilation /#:~:text=Cellars%2C%20attics%20and%20make%2Ddo,from%20 these%20miserable%20living%20conditions.

22   For a detailed description of cholera outbreaks in the United States in these years, see Charles E. Rosenberg, *The Cholera Years: The United States in 1832, 1849, and 1866* (Chicago: University of Chicago Press, 2009).

23   Megan Dunlevy, "Cholera and the Queen City," The Irish in Cincinnati, University of Cincinnati, 2022, libapps.libraries.uc.edu/exhibits/irish -cincinnati/cincinnati-irish-births-and-deaths/cholera-and-the-queen -city/#:~:text=Due%20to%20poor%20living%20conditions,presumably %20brought%20over%20from%20Europe.

24   Daly, "Black Cholera," 143.

25   Anastasia A. Asantewaa, Alex Odoom, Godfred Owusu-Okyere, and Eric S. Donkor, "Cholera Outbreaks in Low- and Middle-Income Countries in the Last Decade: A Systematic Review and Meta-Analysis," *Microorganisms* 12, no. 12 (2024): 2504; Mohammad Ali et al., "The Global Burden of Cholera," *Bulletin of the World Health Organization* 90, no. 3 (2012): 209–18.

26   Several studies document the relationship between cholera and armed conflict. See, for example, Gina E.C. Charnley et al., "Association Between Conflict and Cholera in Nigeria and the Democratic Republic of the Congo," *Emerging Infectious Diseases* 28, no. 12 (2022): 2472; Frederik Federspiel and Mohammad Ali, "The Cholera Outbreak in Yemen: Lessons Learned and Way Forward," *BMC Public Health* 18, no. 1 (2018): 1338; Yousif Ali, Emmanuel Edwar Siddig, and Ayman Ahmed, "Resurgence of Cholera Amidst Ongoing War in Sudan," *The Lancet* 404, no. 10464 (2024): 1724–25; Orwa Al-Abdulla and Maher Alaref, "The Forgotten Threat of Cholera in Syria," *Journal of Water and Health* 20, no. 12 (2022): 1755–60.

27   Amnesty International, "Yemen: Multibillion-Dollar Arms Sales by USA and UK Reveal Shameful Contradiction with Aid Efforts," March 23, 2017, www.amnesty.org/en/latest/news/2017/03/yemen-multibillion-dollar -arms-sales-by-usa-and-uk-reveal-shameful-contradiction-with-aid-efforts. Also see European Center for Constitutional and Human Rights, "Made in Europe, Bombed in Yemen," www.ecchr.eu/en/case/made-in-europe

-bombed-in-yemen/; David Craig, "War Atrocities in Yemen Linked to US Weapons," *Columbia Magazine* (Fall 2022), magazine.columbia.edu/article/war-atrocities-yemen-linked-us-weapons.

28   Christine Crudo Blackburn, Paul E. Lenze, and Rachel Paige Casey, "Conflict and Cholera: Yemen's Man-Made Public Health Crisis and the Global Implications of Weaponizing Health," *Health Security* 18, no. 2 (2020): 125–31.

29   International Rescue Committee, "Yemen Hits 1 Million Cases of Cholera as Even More Preventable Diseases Wreak Havoc on Yemeni Children," press release, December 21, 2017, www.rescue.org/press-release/yemen-hits-1-million-cases-cholera-even-more-preventable-diseases-wreak-havoc-yemeni.

30   United Nations, "Lack of Funds Forces UN to Close Down Life-Saving Aid Programmes in Yemen," August 21, 2019, news.un.org/en/story/2019/08/1044681.

31   Frederik Federspiel and Mohammad Ali, "The Cholera Outbreak in Yemen: Lessons Learned and Way Forward," *BMC Public Health* 18, no. 1 (2018): 1338.

32   Blackburn, Lenze, and Casey, "Conflict and Cholera," 125–31.

33   Save the Children, "Yemen: Cholera Outbreak, 600,000 Children Infected by Christmas," Save the Children, www.savethechildren.org.uk/news/media-centre/press-releases/yemen--cholera-outbreak-now-largest-and-fastest-on-record--600-0.

34   Amnesty International, "Yemen: Multibillion-Dollar Arms Sales by USA and UK Reveal Shameful Contradiction with Aid Efforts," March 23, 2017. https://www.amnesty.org/en/latest/news/2017/03/yemen-multibillion-dollar-arms-sales-by-usa-and-uk-reveal-shameful-contradiction-with-aid-efforts/; also see European Center for Constitutional and Human Rights, "Made in Europe, Bombed in Yemen," https://www.ecchr.eu/en/case/made-in-europe-bombed-in-yemen/; also see David Craig, Fall 2022 issue of *Columbia Magazine*, "War Atrocities in Yemen Linked to US Weapons," https://magazine.columbia.edu/article/war-atrocities-yemen-linked-us-weapons.

35   Mark Landler and Peter Baker, "Trump Vetoes Measure to Force End to U.S. Involvement in Yemen War," *New York Times*, April 16, 2019.

36   Karen DeYoung, "U.S. Restarts Offensive Weapons Sales to Saudi Arabia After Lengthy Ban," *Washington Post*, August 9, 2024.

37   Nasser Abdulkareem, "Yemen: Funding Cuts and Escalation Threaten Peace Prospects and Recovery After Nine Years of Crisis," Norwegian Refugee Council, May 3, 2024, www.nrc.no/perspectives/2024/funding-cuts-leave-yemenis-facing-difficult-choices.

38   "Yemen Humanitarian Update: Issue 3," United Nations Office for the Coordination of Humanitarian Affairs, April 2024, www.unocha.org

/publications/report/yemen/yemen-humanitarian-update-issue-3-april-2024-enar.

39 Wael Bazzi et al., "Heavy Metal Toxicity in Armed Conflicts Potentiates AMR in A. Baumannii by Selecting for Antibiotic and Heavy Metal Co-Resistance Mechanisms," *Frontiers in Microbiology*, no. 11 (2020): 68.

40 There is a large body of research on cholera in Haiti in the aftermath of the earthquake. For example, see Renaud Piarroux et al., "Understanding the Cholera Epidemic, Haiti," *Emerging Infectious Diseases* 17, no. 7 (2011): 1161; Chen-Shan Chin et al., "The Origin of the Haitian Cholera Outbreak Strain," *New England Journal of Medicine* 364, no. 1 (2011): 33–42; John Zarocostas, "Cholera Outbreak in Haiti—from 2010 to Today," *The Lancet* 389, no. 10086 (2017): 2274–75. Also see Paul Farmer's book on the racial and social injustice in Haiti, *Haiti After the Earthquake* (New York: Public Affairs, 2012).

41 "Haiti Significant Earthquake Information," National Oceanic and Atmospheric Administration, www.ngdc.noaa.gov/hazel/view/hazards/earthquake/event-more-info/8732.

42 Reginald DesRoches et al., "Overview of the 2010 Haiti Earthquake," *Earthquake Spectra* 27, no. 1_suppl1 (2011): 1–21.

43 Haiti Significant Earthquake Information available on NOAA US government website, https://www.ngdc.noaa.gov/hazel/view/hazards/earthquake/event-more-info/8732.

44 Iqbal Riza, "Obituary Hedi Annabi," *The Guardian*, January 17, 2010.

45 "Security Council Authorizes 3,500 More UN Peacekeepers for Haiti," UN News, January 19, 2010, news.un.org/en/story/2010/01/326922.

46 "Peacekeeping Without Accountability: The United Nations' Responsibility for the Haitian Cholera Epidemic," Yale Law School, law.yale.edu/sites/default/files/documents/pdf/Clinics/Haiti_TDC_Final_Report.pdf.

47 Daniele Lantagne, G. Balakrish Nair, Claudio F. Lanata, and Alejandro Cravioto, "The Cholera Outbreak in Haiti: Where and How Did It Begin?," in *Cholera Outbreaks* (Berlin: Springer Berlin Heidelberg, 2013), 145–64.

48 Rene S. Hendriksen et al., "Population Genetics of *Vibrio cholerae* from Nepal In 2010: Evidence on the Origin of the Haitian Outbreak," *mBio* 2, no. 4 (2011): 10–11.

49 Anna Lena Lopez et al., "Cholera in Selected Countries in Asia," *Vaccine* 38 (2020): A18–A24.

50 "Haiti Cholera Outbreak: Nepal Troops Not Tested," *BBC News* South Asia, December 8, 2010, www.bbc. co.uk/news/world-south-asia-11949181.

51 Joseph A. Lewnard et al., "Strategies to Prevent Cholera Introduction During International Personnel Deployments: A Computational Modeling Analysis Based on the 2010 Haiti Outbreak," *PLOS Medicine* 13, no. 1 (2016): e1001947.

52   Ref 53. "Haiti Cholera Outbreak: Nepal Troops Not Tested," *BBC News South Asia*, December 8, 2010, www.bbc. co.uk/news/world-south-asia -11949181.

53   "Peacekeeping Without Accountability."

54   Ibid.

55   Ibid.

56   Ibid.

57   Jemima Pierre, "Cholera, Colonization, and the UN's Militarized Humanitarianism in Haiti," *Society for Cultural Anthropology*, January 25, 2022, culanth.org/fieldsights/cholera-colonization-and-the-uns-militarized -humanitarianism-in-haiti#:~:text=The%20cholera%20epidemic%20 is%20an,Haiti's%20poverty%20and%20unsanitary%20conditions.

58   Ralph R. Frerichs, Paul S. Keim, Robert Barrais, and Renaud Piarroux, "Nepalese Origin of Cholera Epidemic in Haiti," *Clinical Microbiology and Infection* 18, no. 6 (2012): E158–63.

59   Yodeline Guillaume et al., "'It Was a Ravage!': Lived Experiences of Epidemic Cholera in Rural Haiti," *BMJ Global Health* 4, no. 6 (2019): e001834.

60   "Peacekeeping Without Accountability."

61   "Haiti Cholera Outbreak Report," CDC Office of Readiness and Response, October 22, 2010–March 15, 2011, www.cdc.gov/orr/responses/haiti -cholera-outbreak.html.

62   P. Farmer et al., "Meeting Cholera's Challenge to Haiti and the World: A Joint Statement on Cholera Prevention and Care," *PLOS Neglected Tropical Diseases* 5, no. 5 (2011): p.e1145.

63   Liz Mineo, "Forcing the UN to Do Right by Haitian Cholera Victims," *Harvard Gazette*, October 6, 2020, news.harvard.edu/gazette/story/2020 /10/a-decade-of-seeking-justice-for-haitian-cholera-victims.

64   *Violations of the Right to Effective Remedy: The UN's Responsibility for Cholera in Haiti*, Joint Submission to the UN Special Rapporteur on the Promotion of Truth, Justice, Reparation and Guarantees of Non-Recurrence, www.ijdh.org/wp-content/uploads/2020/02/FINAL -HLS-IHRC-IJDH-BAI-Submission-to-Special-Procedures-Cholera-2 -6-2020.pdf.

65   Richard Weinmeyer, "Pursuing Justice in Haiti's Cholera Epidemic," *AMA Journal of Ethics* 18, no. 7 (2016): 178–26.

66   "Haiti Cholera Victims' Compensation Claims 'Not Receivable' Under Immunities and Privileges Convention, United Nations Tells Their Representatives," UN News, February 21, 2013, press.un.org/en/2013/sgsm 14828.doc.htm.

67   Rashmee Roshan and Lall Ed Pilkington, "UN Will Not Compensate Haiti Cholera Victims, Ban Ki-Moon Tells President," *The Guardian*, February 21, 2013, www.theguardian.com/world/2013/feb/21/un-haiti -cholera-victims-rejects-compensation.

68 "Secretary-General Apologizes for United Nations Role in Haiti Cholera Epidemic, Urges International Funding of New Response to Disease," UN News press release, December 1, 2016, press.un.org/en/2016/sgsm18323.doc.htm.

69 Ed Pilkington and Ben Quinn, "UN Admits for First Time That Peacekeepers Brought Cholera to Haiti," *The Guardian*, December 1, 2016, www.theguardian.com/global-development/2016/dec/01/haiti-cholera-outbreak-stain-on-reputation-un-says.

70 Ibid.

71 Ed Pilkington, "UN Response to Haiti Cholera Epidemic Lambasted By Its Own Rights Monitors," *The Guardian*, May 4, 2020, www.theguardian.com/world/2020/may/04/united-nations-un-haiti-cholera-letter-rights-monitors.

72 Anastasia Maloney, "A Decade After U.N.-Linked Cholera Outbreak, Haitians Demand Justice," Reuters, October 22, 2020, www.reuters.com/article/world/a-decade-after-un-linked-cholera-outbreak-haitians-demand-justice-idUSKBN2772RL.

73 Pilkington, "UN Response."

74 Ibid.

75 Widlore Merancourt and Amanda Coletta, "The U.N. Is Mulling Another Mission to Haiti. Haitians Are Skeptical," *Washington Post*, November 12, 2022, www.washingtonpost.com/world/2022/11/12/haiti-cholera-united-nations.

76 Ibid.

77 Ibid.

5. The Living Lab

1 "French Doctor Apologizes for Suggesting COVID-19 Treatment Be Tested in Africa," Reuters, April 3, 2020, www.reuters.com/article/world/french-doctor-apologises-for-suggesting-covid-19-treatment-be-tested-in-africa-idUSKBN21L2MR.

2 "Coronavirus: Africa Will Not Be Testing Ground for Vaccine, Says WHO," *BBC News*, April 6, 2020, www.bbc.com/news/world-africa-52192184.

3 Helen Tilley, "Medicine, Empires, and Ethics in Colonial Africa," *AMA Journal of Ethics* 18, no. 7 (2016): 743–53.

4 Samuel Coghe, "Disease Control and Public Health in Colonial Africa," in *Oxford Research Encyclopedia of African History*, November 19, 2020, doi.org/10.1093/acrefore/9780190277734.013.620.

5 Ann Beck, "The Role of Medicine in German East Africa," *Bulletin of the History of Medicine* 45, no. 2 (1971): 170–78.

6 "Trypanosomiasis, Human African (Sleeping Sickness)," WHO, May 2, 2023, www.who.int/news-room/fact-sheets/detail/trypanosomiasis-human-african-(sleeping-sickness).

7   Dietmar Steverding, "The History of African Trypanosomiasis," *Parasites and Vectors*, no. 1 (2008): 1–8.

8   Ian Maudlin, "African Trypanosomiasis," *Annals of Tropical Medicine and Parasitology* 100, no. 8 (2006): 679–701.

9   Mari K. Webel, *The Politics of Disease Control: Sleeping Sickness in Eastern Africa, 1890–1920* (Athens: Ohio University Press, 2019).

10   Lea Berrang-Ford et al., "Sleeping Sickness in Uganda: Revisiting Current and Historical Distributions," *African Health Sciences* 6, no. 4 (2006).

11   Keely Collins, "Deconstructing Memories of Modern Medical Heroes: Robert Koch and the Bugalla Sleeping Sickness Camp, 1900–1910" (PhD diss., University of Victoria, 2023).

12   Editorial, "The Prophylaxis of Sleeping Sickness," *The Lancet*, 2 (July 14, 1906): 101–2.

13   Keely Collins, "Deconstructing Memories of Modern Medical Heroes: Robert Koch and the Bugalla Sleeping Sickness Camp, 1900–1910."

14   Wolfgang U. Eckart, "The Colony as Laboratory: German Sleeping Sickness Campaigns in German East Africa and in Togo, 1900–1914," *History and Philosophy of the Life Sciences* (2002): 69–89.

15   For a discussion of Koch's role, see Collins, "Deconstructing Memories of Modern Medical Heroes: Robert Koch and the Bugalla Sleeping Sickness Camp, 1900–1910" and "The Colony as Laboratory: German Sleeping Sickness Campaigns in German East Africa and in Togo, 1900–1914," *History and Philosophy of the Life Sciences* (2002): 69–89.

16   Christoph Gradmann, "Robert Koch and the Pressures of Scientific Research: Tuberculosis and Tuberculin," *Medical History* 45, no. 1 (2001): 1–32; Donatella Lippi, and Eduardo Gotuzzo, "The Greatest Steps Towards the Discovery of *Vibrio cholerae*," *Clinical Microbiology and Infection* 20, no. 3 (2014): 191–95.

17   Muhammad Hamid Zaman, *Biography of Resistance* (New York: Harper-Collins, 2020).

18   Nobuo Okui, "Shibasaburo Kitasato (1853–1931): Pioneer of Japanese Medicine and Global Immunology Innovator," *Cureus* 16, no. 8 (2024): e68276.

19   Gian Franco Gensini, Andrea Alberto Conti, and Donatella Lippi, "The Contributions of Paul Ehrlich to Infectious Disease," *Journal of Infection* 54, no. 3 (2007): 221–24.

20   Florian Winau, Otto Westphal, and Rolf Winau, "Paul Ehrlich—In Search of the Magic Bullet," *Microbes and Infection* 6, no. 8 (2004): 786–89.

21   Collins, "Deconstructing Memories of Modern Medical Heroes: Robert Koch and the Bugalla Sleeping Sickness Camp, 1900–1910."

22   Eckart, "Colony as Laboratory," 69–89.

23   Rubert Boyce, "The Treatment of Sleeping Sickness and Other Trypanosomiases by the Atoxyl and Mercury Method," *British Medical Journal* 2, no. 2437 (1907): 624.

24   F. Loeffler and K. Riihs, "The Cure of Experimental Nagana (Tsetse Disease)," *Deutsche Medizinische Wochenschrift* 33, no. 34 (1907): 1362.

25   Eckart, "Colony as Laboratory," 69–89.

26   "News in Brief," *The Times*, December 17, 1906, 6.

27   Webel, *Politics of Disease Control*.

28   Collins, "Deconstructing Memories." See also Manuela Bauche, "Robert Koch, Sleeping Sickness and Human Experiments in Colonial East Africa," Freiburg Postkolonial, www.freiburg-postkolonial.de/Seiten/robertkoch. htm.

29   Eckart, "Colony as Laboratory," 69–89.

30   "News in Brief," *The Times*, December 17, 1906, 6.

31   Robert Koch, "Final Report on the Activities of the German Expedition for Research into Sleeping Sickness," *Deutsche Medizinische Wochenschrift* 46 (April 25, 1907): 536.

32   Loeffler and Riihs, "The Cure of Experimental Nagana (Tsetse Disease)," 1362.

33   Eckart, "Colony as Laboratory," 69–89.

34   F.K. Kleine, *Ein deutscher Tropenarzt* (Hannover: Schmorl and von Seefeld, 1949).

35   Robert Koch, "SchluBbericht iiber die Tatigkeit der deutschen Expedition zur Erforschung der Schlafkrankheit," in [Koch's] *Gesammelte Werke*, vol. 2, part 1, ed. J. Schwalbe (Leipzig: Thieme, 1912), 534–46.

36   Dietmar Steverding, "The History of African Trypanosomiasis," *Parasites and Vectors*, no. 1 (2008): 1–8; Harry P. De Koning, "The Drugs of Sleeping Sickness: Their Mechanisms of Action and Resistance, and a Brief History," *Tropical Medicine and Infectious Disease* 5, no. 1 (2020): 14.

37   Koch, "Final Report," 536.

38   Ibid.

39   Eckart, "Colony as Laboratory," 69–89.

40   For a history of the Boer concentration camps, see Elizabeth Van Heyningen, *The Concentration Camps of the Anglo-Boer War: A Social History* (Auckland Park: Jacana Media, 2013).

41   Eckart, "Colony as Laboratory," 69–89.

42   "Dr. Friedrich Karl Kleine," S2A3 Biographical Database of Southern African Science, www.s2a3.org.za/bio/Biograph_final.php?serial=1548.

43   Eckart, "Colony as Laboratory," 69–89.

44   F.K. Kleine, *Medizinal-Berichte iiber die Oeutschen Schutzgebiete fiir das Jahr*, 1911a, 1908/1909.

45   Ibid.

46   Ibid.

47   Dennis Laumann, "A Historiography of German Togoland, or the Rise and Fall of a 'Model Colony,'" *History in Africa* 30 (2003): 195–211.

48   Daniel Glenn Underwood, "Come Hell, or High Water: Tropical Doctors, Sleeping Sickness, and German Colonialism in Togo, Cameroon,

and East Africa 1901–1914 (master's thesis, University of North Carolina at Charlotte, 2024).

49   Eckart, "Colony as Laboratory," 69–89.

50   Patrick Malloy, "Research Material and Necromancy: Imagining the Political-Economy of Biomedicine in Colonial Tanganyika," *International Journal of African Historical Studies* 47, no. 3 (2014): 425–43.

51   Eckart, "Colony as Laboratory," 69–89.

52   Ibid.

53   Ibid.

54   *Denkschrift über die Entwicklung der Schutzgebiete in Afrika und der Südsee im Jahre 1908/09*, Verhandlungen des Reichstags, Sten. Ber. 271 (1911).

55   Eckart, "Colony as Laboratory," 69–89.

56   M. Zupitza, "Tatigkeit der Schlafkrankheitskommission," in *Medizinal-Berichte uber die Deutschen Schutzgebiete fur das Jahr 1908/09* (Berlin, 1911), 292–313.

57   Eckart, "Colony as Laboratory," 69–89.

58   Ibid.

59   Zupitza, "Tatigkeit der Schlafkrankheitskommission."

60   Eckart, "Colony as Laboratory," 69–89.

61   Ibid.

62   Ibid.

63   Underwood, "Come Hell, or High Water."

64   Collins, "Deconstructing Memories."

6. WE SHORTENED THEIR LIVES

1   Martin J. Tobin, "Fiftieth Anniversary of Uncovering the Tuskegee Syphilis Study: The Story and Timeless Lessons," *American Journal of Respiratory and Critical Care Medicine* 205, no. 10 (2022): 1145–58. Note that though I use the spelling of Peter Buxton with an "o" toward the end of his last name, some places spell it as "Buxtun." Both spellings appear in the literature.

2   For a detailed account of the history of the U.S. Public Health Service, see George Rosen, *A History of Public Health* (Baltimore: Johns Hopkins University Press, 2015).

3   John Duffy, *The Sanitarians: A History of American Public Health* (Champaign: University of Illinois Press, 1992).

4   Carl Elliott, "Tuskegee Truth Teller," *American Scholar*, December 4, 2017, theamericanscholar.org/tuskegee-truth-teller.

5   Allen Hornblum, "The Jewish VD Detective Who Exposed the Infamous Tuskegee Experiment," *Tablet Magazine*, January 31, 2021, www.tabletmag .com/sections/history/articles/peter-buxtun-tuskegee-experiment.

6   Elliott, "Tuskegee Truth Teller."

7   Trip Gabriel, "Peter Buxtun, Who Exposed Tuskegee Syphilis Study, Dies at 86," *New York Times*, July 18, 2024.

8   Hornblum, "Jewish VD Detective."

9   Elliott, "Tuskegee Truth Teller."

10   Ibid.

11   Ibid.

12   Hornblum, "Jewish VD Detective."

13   James H. Jones, *Bad Blood: The Tuskegee Syphilis Experiment* (New York: Free Press, 1993).

14   Hornblum, "Jewish VD Detective."

15   Elliott, "Tuskegee Truth Teller."

16   Allen Breed, "How an AP Reporter Broke the Tuskegee Syphilis Story," AP News, July 25, 2022, apnews.com/article/tuskegee-study-experiment -syphilis-7743bd8c7d51fe0ef9a855b4bec69b1f.

17   Ibid.

18   Ibid.

19   Jeroslyn JoVonn, "Reporter Who Exposed the Tuskeegee Experiment Speaks Out 50 Years Later," *Black Enterprise*, July 26, 2022, www .blackenterprise.com/reporter-who-exposed-the-tuskeegee-experiment -speaks-out-50-years-later; Jean Heller and the Associated Press, "Syphilis Victims in U.S. Study Went Untreated for 40 Years," *New York Times*, July 26, 1972, www.nytimes.com/1972/07/26/archives/syphilis-victims -in-us-study-went-untreated-for-40-years-syphilis.html.

20   Dov Ospovat, *The Development of Darwin's Theory: Natural History, Natural Theology, and Natural Selection, 1838–1859* (Cambridge: Cambridge University Press, 1995).

21   Janet Browne, *Darwin's Origin of Species: A Biography* (New York: Grove Press, 1981).

22   Robert G. Perrin, "Herbert Spencer's Four Theories of Social Evolution," *American Journal of Sociology* 81, no. 6 (1976): 1339–59; Gregory Radick, "Darwinism and Social Darwinism," in *The Cambridge History of Modern European Thought*, ed. W. Breckman and P.E. Gordon (Cambridge: Cambridge University Press, 2019), 279–300.

23   Gregory Claeys, "The 'Survival of the Fittest' and the Origins of Social Darwinism," *Journal of the History of Ideas* 61, no. 2 (2000): 223–40.

24   "Sir Francis Galton," Center for the History of Medicine, Harvard University, collections.countway.harvard.edu/onview/exhibits/show/galtons children/sir-francis-galton.

25   Ibid.

26   Paul A. Lombardo and Gregory M. Dorr, "Eugenics, Medical Education, and the Public Health Service: Another Perspective on the Tuskegee Syphilis Experiment," *Bulletin of the History of Medicine* 80, no. 2 (2006): 291–316.

27   William T. English, "The Negro Problem from the Physician's Point of View," *Atlanta Journal-Record of Medicine* 5, no. 461 (1903): 500–01.

28   Daniel K. Shute, "Racial Anatomical Peculiarities," *American Anthropologist* 9, no. 4 (1896): 123–32.

29   Allan M. Brandt, "Racism and Research: The Case of the Tuskegee Syphilis Study," *Hastings Center Report* (1978): 21–29.

30   Daniel David Quillian, "Racial Peculiarities: A Cause of the Prevalence of Syphilis in Negroes," *American Journal of Dermatology and Genito-Urinary Diseases* 10 (1906): 277.

31   Thomas W. Murrell, "Syphilis in the Negro: Its Bearing on the Race Problem," *American Journal of Dermatology and Genito-Urinary Diseases* 10 (1906): 305–6.

32   Thomas G. Benedek and Jonathon Erlen, "The Scientific Environment of the Tuskegee Study of Syphilis, 1920–1960," *Perspectives in Biology and Medicine* 43, no. 1 (1999): 1–30.

33   Anniken Sandvik and Anne Kveim Lie, "Untreated Syphilis: From Oslo to Tuskegee," *Tidsskrift for den Norske laegeforening: tidsskrift for praktisk medicin, ny raekke* 136, no. 23–24 (2016): 2010–16.

34   Brandt, "Racism and Research."

35   Sandvik and Lie, "Untreated Syphilis from Oslo to Tuskegee," *Tidsskrift for den Norske laegeforening: tidsskrift for praktisk medicin, ny raekke* 136, no. 23–24 (2016): 2010–16.

36   Benedek and Erlen, "Scientific Environment," 35–50.

37   Susan M. Reverby, *Examining Tuskegee: The Infamous Syphilis Study and Its Legacy* (Chapel Hill: University of North Carolina Press, 2009).

38   Lisa Ekselius, Bengt Gerdin, and Anders Vahlquist, "The Syphilis Pandemic Prior to Penicillin: Origin, Health Issues, Cultural Representation and Ethical Challenges," *Acta Dermato-venereologica*, no. 104 (2024).

39   Mircea Tampa et al., "Brief History of Syphilis," *Journal of Medicine and Life* 7, no. 1 (2014): 4.

40   P. Hemarajata, "A Brief History of Laboratory Diagnostics for Syphilis," *ASM Org*, 2020.

41   Gian Franco Gensini, Andrea Alberto Conti, and Donatella Lippi, "The Contributions of Paul Ehrlich to Infectious Disease," *Journal of Infection* 54, no. 3 (2007): 221–24.

42   Henry J. Nichols and John A. Fordyce, "The Treatment of Syphilis with Ehrlich's 606," *Journal of the American Medical Association* 55, no. 14 (1910): 1171–78.

43   John Parascandola, "History of Salvarsan (Arsphenamine)," *Chemotherapy* 32 (2001): 151–71.

44   R.W. Kapp, "Arsenic: Toxicology and Health Effects," in *Encyclopedia of Food and Health* (New York: Academic Press, 2016), 256–65.

45   Brandt, "Racism and Research," 21–29.

46   Joseph E. Moore, *The Modern Treatment of Syphilis* (Baltimore: Charles C. Thomas, 1933).

47   Brandt, "Racism and Research," 21–29.

48   Reverby, *Examining Tuskegee.*

49   Ibid.

50   Robert M. White, "Unraveling the Tuskegee Study of Untreated Syphilis," *Archives of Internal Medicine* 160, no. 5 (2000): 585–98.

51   Brandt, "Racism and Research," 21–29.

52   Brandt, "Racism and Research," 21–29; Martin J. Tobin, "Fiftieth Anniversary of Uncovering the Tuskegee Syphilis Study: The Story and Timeless Lessons," *American Journal of Respiratory and Critical Care Medicine* 205, no. 10 (2022): 1145–58.

53   Allen Hornblum, "The Secret Story of How a Revered Future Surgeon General Inspired the Tuskegee Syphilis Study," *Daily Beast*, August 19, 2017.

54   "Race May Be Cause of Negro's Lower Tuberculosis Resistance," *Science News-Letter* 21, no. 585 (1932): 409.

55   Aimee Cunningham, "Medical Racism Didn't Begin or End with the Syphilis Study at Tuskegee," *Science News*, December 20, 2022, www .sciencenews.org/article/tuskegee-syphilis-study-medical-racism.

56   H.S. Cumming to R.R. Morton, September 20, 1932, NA-WNRC.

57   Lombardo and Dorr, "Eugenics."

58   Brandt, "Racism and Research."

59   Brandt, "Racism and Research."

60   Brandt, "Racism and Research."

61   Lombardo and Dorr, "Eugenics."

62   Vonderlehr quoted in Susan L. Smith, *Sick and Tired of Being Sick and Tired: Black Women's Health Activism in America, 1890–1950* (Philadelphia: University of Pennsylvania Press, 1995), 109.

63   The role of Eunice Rivers, a Black nurse, has been debated extensively by historians and public health scholars. For details, see Reverby, *Examining Tuskegee.*

64   Reverby, *Examining Tuskegee.*

65   Brandt, "Racism and Research."

66   Brandt, "Racism and Research."

67   Ibid.

68   Susan Reverby, "Rethinking the Tuskegee Syphilis Study," in *Tuskegee's Truths: Rethinking the Tuskegee Syphilis Study* (Chapel Hill: University of North Carolina Press, 2012), 365.

69   Christopher Crenner, "The Tuskegee Syphilis Study and the Scientific Concept of Racial Nervous Resistance," *Journal of the History of Medicine and Allied Sciences* 67, no. 2 (2012): 244–80.

70   E.M. Hummel, "The Rarity of Tabetic and Paretic Conditions in the Negro: A Case of Tabes in a Full-Blood Negress," *Journal of the American Medical Association* 56, no. 22 (1911): 1645-1646.

71   Ibid.

72   Brandt, "Racism and Research."

73   Reverby, "Rethinking."

74   Reverby, *Examining Tuskegee.*
75   Ibid.
76   Brandt, "Racism and Research."
77   Reverby, *Examining Tuskegee.*
78   Ibid.
79   O. C. Wenger, in *Tuskegee's Truths: Rethinking the Tuskegee Syphilis Study*, ed. S. M. Reverby (Chapel Hill: University of North Carolina Press, 2000), 84–85.
80   Reverby, *Examining Tuskegee.*
81   Brandt, "Racism and Research."
82   Reverby, *Examining Tuskegee.*
83   Wenger, in *Tuskegee's Truths.*
84   Brandt, "Racism and Research."
85   Reverby, *Examining Tuskegee.*
86   James H. Jones, *Bad Blood: The Tuskegee Syphilis Experiment* (New York: Simon and Schuster, 1993).
87   Susan M. Reverby, "The Milbank memorial fund and the US public health service study of untreated syphilis in Tuskegee: a short historical reassessment," *The Milbank Quarterly* 100, no. 2 (2022): 327.
88   Reverby, "Milbank Memorial Fund."
89   Reverby, *Examining Tuskegee*, 53.
90   Raymond A. Vonderlehr, Taliaferro Clark, Oliver C. Wenger, and J.R. Heller, "Untreated Syphilis in the Male Negro: A Comparative Study of Treated and Untreated Cases," *Journal of the American Medical Association* 107, no. 11 (1936): 856–60.
91   Reverby, *Examining Tuskegee.*
92   Ibid.
93   Christopher Crenner, "The Tuskegee Syphilis Study and the Scientific Concept of Racial Nervous Resistance," *Journal of the History of Medicine and Allied Sciences* 67, no. 2 (2012): 244–80; Reverby, *Examining Tuskegee.*
94   L.V. Stamm, "Syphilis: Antibiotic Treatment and Resistance," *Epidemiology and Infection* 143, no. 8 (2015): 1567–74.
95   Reverby, *Tuskegee's Truths.*
96   Ibid.
97   Brandt, "Racism and Research."
98   Reverby, *Examining Tuskegee.*
99   Ibid.
100   Martin J. Tobin, "Fiftieth Anniversary of Uncovering the Tuskegee Syphilis Study: The Story and Timeless Lessons," *American Journal of Respiratory and Critical Care Medicine* 205, no. 10 (2022): 1145–58.
101   Ibid.
102   Ibid.
103   Jones, *Bad Blood.*

104 See Robert M. White, "Unraveling the Tuskegee Study of Untreated Syphilis," *Archives of Internal Medicine* 160, no. 5 (2000): 585–98; Brandt, "Racism and Research"; Reverby, *Examining Tuskegee.*
105 Rudolph H. Kampmeier, "The Tuskegee Study of Untreated Syphilis," *Southern Medical Journal* 65, no. 10 (1972): 1247–51.
106 Ibid.
107 Joel Howell, "Race and US Medical Experimentation: The Case of Tuskegee," *Cadernos de saude publica* 33, no. Suppl 1 (2017): e00168016.
108 Lynn M. Harter, Ronald J. Stephens, and Phyllis M. Japp, "President Clinton's Apology for the Tuskegee Syphilis Experiment: A Narrative of Remembrance, Redefinition, and Reconciliation," *Howard Journal of Communication* 11, no. 1 (2000): 19–34.
109 Alison Mitchell, "Clinton Regrets 'Clearly Racist' U.S. Study," *New York Times*, May 17, 1997, www.nytimes.com/1997/05/17/us/clinton-regrets-clearly-racist-us-study.html.
110 Ibid.
111 Ibid.

7. You Know, We Couldn't Do Such an Experiment in This Country

1 Lynne Page Snyder, "The Career of Surgeon General Thomas J. Parran, Jr., MD, (1892–1968)," *Public Health Reports* 110, no. 5 (1995): 630.
2 J. David Oriel, "Public Health Matters," in *The Scars of Venus: A History of Venereology* (London: Springer-Verlag, 1994), 191–211.
3 Daniel Sledge, "Linking Public Health and Individual Medicine: The Health Policy Approach of Surgeon General Thomas Parran," *American Journal of Public Health* 107, no. 4 (2017): 509–16.
4 Thomas Parran Jr., "A New Health Program for New York State," *Journal of the American Medical Association* 97, no. 11 (1931): 763–66; Thomas Parran Jr., "Public Medical Care in New York State," *Journal of the American Medical Association* 101, no. 5 (1933): 342–45.
5 Sledge, "Linking Public Health."
6 "Dr. Parran Named Surgeon General; President Nominates State Health Commissioner to Succeed Dr. Hugh S. Cumming," *New York Times*, March 24, 1936, www.nytimes.com/1936/03/24/archives/dr-parran-named-surgeon-general-president-nominates-state-health.html.
7 Thomas Parran, "The Eradication of Syphilis as a Practical Public Health Objective," *Journal of the American Medical Association* 97, no. 2 (1931): 73–77.
8 "Medicine, Syphilis and Radio," *Time*, December 3, 1934, time.com/archive/6863262/medicine-syphilis-radio.
9 George H. Ramsey, "Review of *Shadow on the Land: Syphilis* by Thomas Parran," *Milbank Memorial Fund Quarterly* 16, no. 1 (January 1938): 108–10;

Kenneth A. Katz, "Congenital Syphilis—Still a Shadow on the Land," *JAMA Dermatology* 154, no. 12 (2018): 1389–90.

10   James H. Jones, *Bad Blood: The Tuskegee Syphilis Experiment* (New York: Free Press, 1993), 58, 67.

11   William Bender, "Did a U.S. Surgeon General Come Up with the Idea of the Notorious Tuskegee Syphilis Experiment?," *Philadelphia Inquirer*, www .inquirer.com/philly/news/thomas-parran-tuskegee-syphilis-hornblum -experiment-20170720.html; "Public Health Symposium Panelists Discuss Legacy of Parran Hall Namesake," *University Times* (University of Pittsburgh), April 11, 2018, www.utimes.pitt.edu/news/public-health -symposium.

12   Susan M. Reverby, ed., *Tuskegee's Truths: Rethinking the Tuskegee Syphilis Study* (Chapel Hill: University of North Carolina Press, 2012).

13   Ibid.

14   Bender, "Did a U.S. Surgeon General."

15   Edward W. Hook III, "Remembering Thomas Parran, His Contributions and Missteps Going Forward: History Informs Us," *Sexually Transmitted Diseases* 40, no. 4 (2013): 281–82.

16   Joseph Moore to A.N. Richards. (1943, February 1), Correspondence. PCSBI HSPI Archives, NARA-II_0000176.

17   John A. Rogers to Lewis H. Weed. (1942, December 4). Correspondence. PCSBI HSPI Archives, NARA-II_0000283.

18   Evan W. Thomas, "John F. Mahoney, MD, 1889–1957," *AMA Archives of Dermatology* 76, no. 1 (1957): 118.

19   Ibid.

20   Jan Ackerman and *Post-Gazette* Staff Writer, "Obituary: John Charles Cutler/Pioneer in Preventing Sexual Diseases," *Pittsburgh Post-Gazette* 12 (2003): 144–51.

21   Matthew Walter, "First, Do Harm," *Nature* 482, no. 7384 (2012): 148–52.

22   Sushma Subramanian, "Worse than Tuskegee," *Slate*, February 26, 2017, www.slate.com/articles/health_and_science/cover_story/2017/02 /guatemala_syphilis_experiments_worse_than_tuskegee.html; Donald McNeil, "Panel Hears Grim Details of Venereal Disease Tests," *New York Times*, August 30, 2011.

23   Susan M. Reverby, "'Normal Exposure' and Inoculation Syphilis: A PHS 'Tuskegee' Doctor in Guatemala, 1946–1948," *Journal of Policy History* 23, no. 1 (2011): 6–28.

24   Subramanian, "Worse than Tuskegee."

25   Ivan Semeniuk, "A Shocking Discovery," *Nature* 467, no. 7316 (2010): 645; Matthew, "First, Do Harm."

26   Subramanian, "Worse than Tuskegee."

27   Kayte Spector-Bagdady and Paul A. Lombardo, "'Something of an Adventure': Postwar NIH Research Ethos and the Guatemala STD Experiments," *Journal of Law, Medicine and Ethics* 41, no. 3 (2013): 697–710.

28   Presidential Commission for the Study of Bioethical Issues, *"Ethically Impossible": STD Research in Guatemala from 1946 to 1948*, 2011, https://law.stanford.edu/wp-content/uploads/2011/09/EthicallyImpossible_PCSBI_110913.pdf.

29   Subramanian, "Worse than Tuskegee."

30   Presidential Commission, *"Ethically Impossible."*

31   Subramanian, "Worse than Tuskegee."

32   Ibid.

33   Presidential Commission, *"Ethically Impossible."*

34   See papers of Dr. Cutler and correspondence in United States. Presidential Commission for the Study of Bioethical Issues, *"Ethically Impossible": STD Research in Guatemala from 1946 to 1948.*

35   Subramanian, "Worse than Tuskegee."

36   Presidential Commission, *"Ethically Impossible."*

37   Ibid.

38   Ibid.

39   Reverby, "'Normal Exposure.'"

40   Jonathan Zenilman, "The Guatemala Sexually Transmitted Disease Studies: What Happened," *Sexually Transmitted Diseases* 40, no. 4 (2013): 277–79.

41   Subramanian, "Worse than Tuskegee."

42   Zenilman, "Guatemala Sexually Transmitted Disease Studies."

43   Presidential Commission, *"Ethically Impossible."*

44   W. Kaempffert, "Notes on Science: Syphilis Prevention," *New York Times*, April 27, 1947.

45   John Cutler to John Mahoney. (1947, May 17). Correspondence. PCSBI HSPI Archives, CTLR_0001122.

46   John Cutler to John Mahoney. (1948, June 22). Correspondence. PCSBI HSPI Archives, CTLR_0001144.

47   *Information on the 1946–1948 United States Public Health Service STD Inoculation Study.* U.S. Department of Health and Human Services.

48   John Mahoney to John Cutler. (1946, October 15). Correspondence. PCSBI HSPI Archives, CTLR_0001200.

49   Paul A. Lombardo and Gregory M. Dorr, "Eugenics, Medical Education, and the Public Health Service: Another Perspective on the Tuskegee Syphilis Experiment," *Bulletin of the History of Medicine* 80, no. 2 (2006): 291–316.

50   CDC Report on Findings from the U.S. Public Health Service Sexually Transmitted Disease Inoculation Study of 1946–1948, based on review of Archived Papers of John Cutler, MD, at the University of Pittsburgh.

51   G. Robert Coatney to John Cutler. (1947, February 17). Correspondence. PCSBI HSPI Archives, CTLR_0001051.

52 John Mahoney to John Cutler. (1948, February 19). Correspondence. PCSBI HSPI Archives, CTLR_0001223.

53 Ibid.

54 Ibid.

55 Personal communication with author, February 2024.

56 See Wellesley College website, www1.wellesley.edu/wgst/faculty/reverby.

57 Personal communication with author, February 2024.

58 "Researcher 'Floored' by Discovery of Intentional Infections in Guatemala," PBS interview of Dr. Reverby, October 4, 2010, www.pbs.org/newshour/show/researcher-floored-by-discovery-of-intentional-infections-in-guatemala.

59 "Historian's Research at Pitt Prompts Presidential Apology," *University Times* (University of Pittsburgh), March 31, 2011, www.utimes.pitt.edu/archives/?p=15854.

60 Susan M. Reverby, "Restorative Justice and Restorative History for the Sexually Transmitted Disease Inoculation Experiments in Guatemala," *American Journal of Public Health* 106, no. 7 (2016): 1163.

61 "Historian's Research at Pitt."

62 "Joint Statement by Secretaries Clinton and Sebelius on a 1946–1948 Study," U.S. Department of State, October 1, 2010, 2009-2017.state.gov/secretary/20092013clinton/rm/2010/10/148464.htm.

63 "Read-out of the President's Call with Guatemalan President Colom," The White House, Office of the Press Secretary, October 1, 2010, obamawhitehouse.archives.gov/the-press-office/2010/10/01/read-out-presidents-call-with-guatemalan-president-colom.

64 Presidential Commission, *"Ethically Impossible."*

65 Oliver Laughland, "Guatemalans Deliberately Infected with STDs Sue Johns Hopkins University for $1bn," *The Guardian*, April 2, 2015, www.theguardian.com/us-news/2015/apr/02/johns-hopkins-lawsuit-deliberate-std-infections-guatemala.

66 Paul A. Lombardo, "Victims Again: Litigation Ends on the US Public Health Service Syphilis Studies in Guatemala," *Voices in Bioethics*, no. 10 (2024).

67 "Penicillin as a Cure for Syphilis," 1946 Albert Lasker Clinical Medical Research Award, laskerfoundation.org/winners/penicillin-as-a-cure-for-syphilis.

68 Evan W. Thomas, "John F. Mahoney, MD, 1889–1957," *AMA Archives of Dermatology* 76, no. 1 (1957): 118.

69 Sledge, "Linking Public Health."

70 "Public Health Symposium Panelists Discuss Legacy of Parran Hall Namesake," *University Times* (University of Pittsburgh), April 11, 2018, www.utimes.pitt.edu/news/public-health-symposium.

71 Ibid.

72 Hook, "Remembering Thomas Parran."

73 "Parran Hall Name Disappears After Board of Trustees Agrees with Chancellor's Recommendation," *University Times* (University of Pittsburgh), July 5, 2018, www.utimes.pitt.edu/news/parran-hall-name.

74 Scott Jashik, "Ending Honor for Disgraced Scientist," *Inside Higher Education*, June 28, 2018, www.insidehighered.com/news/2018/06/29/pitt-moves -rename-building-public-health-school-which-honors-disgraced-scientist.

75 Harold J. Magnuson et al., "Inoculation Syphilis in Human Volunteers," *Medicine* 35, no. 1 (1956): 33–82; Reverby, "'Normal Exposure.'"

76 Reverby, "'Normal Exposure.'"

77 Allan M. Brandt, "Racism and Research: The Case of the Tuskegee Syphilis Study," *Hastings Center Report* (1978): 21–29.

78 Donald McNeil, "Panel Hears Grim Details of Venereal Disease Tests," *New York Times*, August 30, 2011, www.nytimes.com/2011/08/31/world /americas/31syphilis.html.

79 Susan M. Reverby, *Examining Tuskegee: The Infamous Syphilis Study and Its Legacy* (Chapel Hill: University of North Carolina Press, 2009).

80 Ibid.

81 Ibid.

82 Ibid.

83 Jan Ackerman, "Obituary: John Charles Cutler, Pioneer in Preventing Sexual Diseases," *Pittsburgh Post-Gazette*, February 12, 2003

84 Ibid.

8. Bacteria as a Bomb

1 Peter Li, ed., "Japan's Biochemical Warfare and Experimentation in China," in *Japanese War Crimes* (London: Routledge, 2017), 289–300. Also note that academic literature uses both Heilongjian and Heilongjiang spellings.

2 Peter Williams and David Wallace, *Unit 731: Japan's Secret Biological Warfare in World War II* (New York: Free Press, 1989).

3 Ibid.

4 Hal Gold, *Unit 731 Testimony: Japan's Wartime Human Experimentation Program* (North Clarendon, VT: Tuttle, 2004); Gregory Dean Byrd, "General Shirō Ishii: His Legacy Is That of Genius and Madman" (master's thesis, East Tennessee State University, 2005), dc.etsu.edu/etd/1010.

5 Ibid.

6 Ibid.

7 Ibid.

8 Ibid.

9 Sheldon H. Harris, *Factories of Death: Japanese Biological Warfare, 1932–45, and the American Cover-Up* (London: Routledge, 1995).

10 Yang Yan-Jun and Tam Yue-Him, *Unit 731: Laboratory of the Devil, Auschwitz of the East: Japanese Biological Warfare in China 1933-45* (Charleston, SC: Fonthill Media, 2018); Byrd, "General Shirō Ishii."

11   Takashi Tsuchiya, "Why Japanese Doctors Performed Human Experiments in China 1933–1945," *Eubios Journal of Asian and International Bioethics* 10, no. 6 (2000).

12   Sophie Hammond, "The Experiments of Unit 731: Torture in the Name of Warfare," Pacific Atrocities Education, June 13, 2018, www.pacific atrocities.org/blog/the-experiments-of-unit-731-torture-in-the-name-of -warfare.

13   Tsuneishi Keiichi, *Unit 731 and the Japanese Imperial Army's Biological Warfare Program*, Vol. 25 (London: Routledge, 2010).

14   Ibid.

15   Gold, *Unit 731*.

16   Jeffrey A. Lockwood, "Insects as Weapons of War, Terror, and Torture," *Annual Review of Entomology* 57, no. 1 (2012): 205–27.

17   James M. Wilson and Mari Daniel, "Historical Reconstruction of the Community Response, and Related Epidemiology, of a Suspected Biological Weapon Attack in Ningbo, China (1940)," *Intelligence and National Security* 34, no. 2 (2019): 278–88.

18   Gold, *Unit 731*.

19   Ibid.

20   Takashi Tsuchiya, "The Imperial Japanese Experiments in China," *The Oxford Textbook of Clinical Research Ethics* (2008): 31–45.

21   Douglas R. Bacon, "Biological Warfare: An Historical Perspective," in *Seminars in Anesthesia, Perioperative Medicine and Pain* 22, no. 4 (December 2003): 224–29.

22   George W. Christopher et al., "Biological Warfare: A Historical Perspective," *Journal of the American Medical Association* 278, no. 5 (August 1997): 412–17.

23   Samuel J. Cox, "H-057-2: I-400 and Operation Cherry Blossoms at Night: Japanese Plan for Biological Warfare—September 1945," Naval History and Heritage Command, January 2021, www.history.navy.mil /about-us/leadership/director/directors-corner/h-grams/h-gram-057/h -057-2.html.

24   Gold, *Unit 731*.

25   Ibid.

26   Jeanne Guillemin, "Scientists and the History of Biological Weapons: A Brief Historical Overview of the Development of Biological Weapons in the Twentieth Century," *EMBO Reports* 7, no. S1 (2006): S45–S49.

27   Ibid.

28   Sheldon H. Harris, *Factories of Death: Japanese Biological Warfare, 1932–45, and the American Cover-Up* (London: Routledge, 1995).

29   The Tokyo tribunals, which were formally called the International Military Tribunal for the Far East (IMTFE), were a series of military trials that started in April 1946 to try leaders of the Empire of Japan for their crimes against humanity. Modeled after the military tribunals in Nuremberg,

these trials lasted until December 1948. Jeanne Guillemin, *Hidden Atrocities: Japanese Germ Warfare and American Obstruction of Justice at the Tokyo Trial* (New York: Columbia University Press, 2017).
30 Guillemin, *Hidden Atrocities.*
31 Ibid.
32 Guillemin, "Scientists."
33 Gold, *Unit 731.*
34 Byrd, "General Shirō Ishii."
35 Nicholas Kristof, "Unmasking Horror: A Special Report; Japan Confronting Gruesome War Atrocity," *New York Times,* March 17, 1995.
36 Jeanne Guillemin, *Biological Weapons: From the Invention of State-Sponsored Programs to Contemporary Bioterrorism* (New York: Columbia University Press, 2005).
37 Ibid.
38 Ibid.
39 Ibid.
40 Frederick O. Banting, "Memorandum on the Present Situation Regarding Bacterial Weapons." *WO188/653* 10 (1939).
41 Guillemin, *Biological Weapons.*
42 Barton J. Bernstein, "America's Biological Warfare Program in the Second World War," *Journal of Strategic Studies* 11, no. 3 (1988): 292–317.
43 Norman Covert, *Cutting Edge: A History of Fort Detrick, Maryland, 1943–1993* (Fort Detrick Headquarters: Public Affairs Office).
44 Guillemin, *Biological Weapons.*
45 Stefan Riedel, "Biological Warfare and Bioterrorism: A Historical Review," in *Baylor University Medical Center Proceedings* 17, no. 4 (2004): 400–406.
46 Guillemin, *Biological Weapons.*
47 Ibid.
48 Barton J. Bernstein, The Birth of the US Biological-Warfare Program," in *Bioterrorism: The History of a Crisis in American Society,* ed. David McBride (New York: Routledge, 2020), 54–59; "The Reclusive Revolutionary: Dr. Elvin Kabat and His Legacy," Columbia University Department of Microbiology and Immunology, microbiology.columbia.edu/dr-elvin-kabat-and-his-legacy-the-reclusive-revolutionary-historical-faculty-highlight.
49 Guillemin, *Biological Weapons.*
50 Ibid.
51 Ibid.
52 Ibid.
53 Ibid.
54 Ibid.
55 Ibid.
56 Ibid.

57   Ibid.
58   Mark G. Kortepeter and Gerald W. Parker, "Potential Biological Weapons Threats," *Emerging Infectious Diseases* 5, no. 4 (1999): 523.
59   Guillemin, *Biological Weapons.*
60   George Sternbach, "The History of Anthrax," *Journal of Emergency Medicine* 24, no. 4 (2003): 463–67; Stefan Riedel, "Anthrax: A Continuing Concern in the Era of Bioterrorism," in *Baylor University Medical Center Proceedings* 18, no. 3 (2005): 234–43.
61   Guillemin, *Biological Weapons.*
62   Ibid.
63   Ibid.
64   Ibid.
65   Anders Sjöstedt, "Tularemia: History, Epidemiology, Pathogen Physiology, and Clinical Manifestations," *Annals of the New York Academy of Sciences* 1105, no. 1 (2007): 1–29.
66   Michael J. Corbel, "Brucellosis: An Overview," *Emerging Infectious Diseases* 3, no. 2 (1997): 213.
67   Hillel W. Cohen, Robert M. Gould, and Victor W. Sidel, "Bioterrorism Initiatives: Public Health in Reverse?," *American Journal of Public Health* 89, no. 11 (1999): 1629–31.
68   Guillemin, *Biological Weapons.*
69   Theodor Rosebury, *Peace or Pestilence? Biological Warfare and How to Avoid It* (New York: Whittlesey House, 1949).
70   Leon J. Warshaw, "Report on Biological Warfare; Peace or Pestilence," ed. Theodor Rosebury (New York: Whittlesey House). *New York Times*, June 5, 1949, www.nytimes.com/1949/06/05/archives/report-on-biological-warfare-peace-or-pestilence-by-theodor.html.
71   National Research Council, "Historical Background of the US Biologic-Warfare Program," in *Toxicologic Assessment of the Army's Zinc Cadmium Sulfide Dispersion Tests* (Washington, DC: National Academies Press, 1997).
72   Guillemin, *Biological Weapons.*
73   Ibid.
74   "Reclusive Revolutionary."
75   Ibid.
76   Ibid.
77   Ibid.
78   Ibid.
79   John Ellis van Courtland Moon, "The US Biological Weapons Program," in *Deadly Cultures: Biological Weapons Since 1945*, ed. Mark Wheelis, Lajos Rózsa, and Malcolm Dando (Cambridge: Harvard University Press, 2006), 9–46.
80   Guillemin, *Biological Weapons.*
81   Ibid.

82 Ibid.

83 Ibid.

84 Moon, "US Biological Weapons Program."

85 Judith Miller, William J. Broad, and Stephen Engelberg, *Germs: Biological Weapons and America's Secret War* (New York: Simon and Schuster, 2012).

86 "Secret Testing in the United States," PBS, The American Experience, www.pbs.org/wgbh/americanexperience/features/weapon-secret-testing.

87 Ibid.

88 "List of Technical Reports at Dugway Proving Ground (DPG) or West Desert Technical Information Center (WDTIC) at Dugway Proving Ground, 1950–1960," www.governmentattic.org/10docs/TechRptsDPG _1950-1960.pdf.

89 U.S. Senate. Committee on Human Resources, Subcommittee on Health and Scientific Research. Biological Testing Involving Human Subjects by the Department of Defense. March 8 and May 23, 1977.

90 Leonard A. Cole, "Open-Air Biowarfare Testing and the Evolution of Values," *Health Security* 14, no. 5 (2016): 315–22.

91 Leonard Cole, "The Worry: Germ Warfare. The Target: Us," *New York Times*, January 25, 1994.

92 Leonard A. Cole, *Clouds of Secrecy: The Army's Germ Warfare Tests over Populated Areas* (Lanham, MD: Rowman and Littlefield, 1988).

93 Alastair Hay, "A Magic Sword or a Big Itch: An Historical Look at the United States Biological Weapons Programme," *Medicine, Conflict and Survival* 15, no. 3 (1999): 215–34.

94 Phillip R. Pittman, Sarah L. Norris, Kevin M. Coonan, and Kelly T. McKee Jr., "An Assessment of Health Status Among Medical Research Volunteers Who Served in the Project Whitecoat Program at Fort Detrick, Maryland," *Military Medicine* 170, no. 3 (2005): 183–87.

95 Guillemin, *Biological Weapons.*

96 CIA records, Memorandum for the Record From L.K. White, www.cia .gov/readingroom/document/cia-rdp80r01284a001800130047-3.

97 Krista Thompson Smith, "Adventists and Biological Warfare," *Spectrum* 25, no. 3 (1996): 35–50.

98 Ibid.

99 Alicia Gutierrez, "Project Operation Whitecoat: Military Experimentation, Seventh-Day Adventism and Conscientious Cooperation," *History in the Making* 3, no. 1 (2010): 6.

100 Mark S. Williams et al., "Retrospective Analysis of Pneumonic Tularemia in Operation Whitecoat Human Subjects: Disease Progression and Tetracycline Efficacy," *Frontiers in Medicine* 6 (2019): 229.

101 Smith, "Adventists and Biological Warfare."

102 Guillemin, *Biological Weapons.*

103 Ibid.

104   Jonathan Moreno, "Secret State Experiments and Medical Ethics," in *Expanding Horizons in Bioethics*, ed. Arthur W. Galston and Christiana Z. Peppard (Dordrecht: Springer Netherlands, 2005), 59–69.

105   "Operation Whitecoat," *Religion and Ethics Newsweekly*, PBS, October 24, 2003, www.pbs.org/wnet/religionandethics/2003/10/24/october -24-2003-operation-whitecoat/15055.

106   Williams et al., "Retrospective Analysis."

107   Gutierrez, "Project Operation Whitecoat."

108   See the perspective of a former volunteer at www.mytripjournal.com /travel-773876-fort-sam-houston-rift-valley-fever-operation-whitecoat.

109   Smith, "Adventists and Biological Warfare."

110   Moon, "US Biological Weapons Program."

111   Brian Balmer and John Ellis van Courtland Moon, "The British, United States and Canadian Biological Warfare Programs," in *Biological Threats in the 21st Century: The Politics, People, Science and Historical Roots*, ed. Filippa Lentzos (London: Imperial College Press, 2016), 43–67.

112   Fact Sheet Office of the Assistant Secretary of Defense, "Yellow Leaf," www.health.mil/Reference-Center/Fact-Sheets/2002/10/31/Yellow -Leaf.

113   Cole, "Open-Air Biowarfare."

114   Guillemin, *Biological Weapons*.

115   Hay, "A Magic Sword."

116   *Survey of Reported Chemical and Biological Contamination at the Fort Greely Gerstle River Test Center*, U.S. Government Accountability Office, November 30, 1979, www.gao.gov/products/lcd-80-25.

117   Steven L. Simon, "A Brief History of People and Events Related to Atomic Weapons Testing in the Marshall Islands," *Health Physics* 73, no. 1 (1997): 5–20.

118   Ibid.

119   Neal A. Palafox, "Health Consequences of the Pacific US Nuclear Weapons Testing Program in the Marshall Islands: Inequity in Protection, Health Care Access, Policy, Regulation," *Reviews on Environmental Health* 25, no. 1 (2010): 81–85.

120   Hearing Before the Subcommittee on Asia the Pacific and the Global Environment of the Committee on Foreign Affairs House of Representatives One Hundred Eleventh Congress, Second Session, May 20, 2010, www .govinfo.gov/content/pkg/CHRG-111hhrg56559/html/CHRG -111hhrg56559.htm.

121   Susanne Rust, "How the US Betrayed the Marshall Islands, Kindling the Next Nuclear Disaster," *Los Angeles Times*, November 10, 2019.

122   Ibid.

123   "Fact Sheet: Project Shipboard Hazard and Defense (SHAD), DTC Test 68–50," Special Assistant to the Under Secretary of Defense (Personnel and Readiness) for Gulf War, Illnesses, Medical Readiness, and Military

Deployments, May 23, 2002, www.health.mil/Reference-Center/Fact
-Sheets/2002/05/23/DTC-Test-6850.

124 Rust, "Kindling the Next Nuclear Disaster."

125 Barbara Rose Johnston, Holly M. Barker, and Bill Graham, *Hardships
and Consequential Damages from Radioactive Contamination, Denied
Use, Exile, and Human Subject Experimentation Experienced by the People
of Rongelap, Rongerik, and Ailinginae Atolls*, Marshall Islands Nuclear
Claims Tribunal Office of the Public Advocate, September 17, 2001.

126 Elizabeth A. Willis, "Landscape with Dead Sheep: What They Did to
Gruinard Island," *Medicine, Conflict and Survival* 25, no. 4 (2009):
320–31.

127 For a short note on the life and work of Roy Vollum, see "Roy Lars Vollum,
M.A. British Columbia and Oxon, D. Phil.," *Lancet* 1, no. 7655 (May 16,
1970): 1065.

128 S.L. Welkos, T.J. Keener, and P.H. Gibbs, "Differences in Susceptibility of
Inbred Mice to *Bacillus anthracis*," *Infection and Immunity* 51, no. 3
(1986): 795–800.

129 Elizabeth A. Willis, "Landscape with Dead Sheep: What They Did to
Gruinard Island," *Medicine, Conflict and Survival* 25, no. 4 (2009):
320–31.

130 Steven Brocklehurst, "The Mystery of Anthrax Island and the Seeds of
Death," *BBC News*, February 26, 2022.

131 Brian Balmer, "Killing Without the Distressing Preliminaries: Scientists'
Defence of the British Biological Warfare Programme," *Minerva* 40,
no. 1 (2002): 57–75.

132 Richard Nixon, "Remarks Announcing Decisions on Chemical and Biological Defense Policies and Programs," November 25, 1969, The American Presidency Project, www.presidency.ucsb.edu/documents/remarks
-announcing-decisions-chemical-and-biological-defense-policies-and
-programs; Milton Leitenberg and Raymond A. Zilinskas, *The Soviet Biological Weapons Program: A History* (Cambridge, MA: Harvard University
Press, 2012).

133 Leitenberg and Zilinskas, *Soviet Biological Weapons Program.*

134 John Hart, "The Soviet Biological Weapons Program," *Deadly Cultures*
(2006): 132–56.

135 Raymond A. Zilinskas, *The Soviet Biological Weapons Program and Its
Legacy in Today's Russia* (Washington, DC: National Defense University Press, 2014).

136 Special Issues Dedicated to the 90th Anniversary of the Founder of the
Journal, Academician of the Russian Academy of Sciences Yuri Anatol'evich
Ovchinnikov, *Russian Journal of Bioorganic Chemistry* 50 (June 2024):
627–28, doi.org/10.1134/S1068162024030075.

137 Anthony Rimmington, *Stalin's Secret Weapon: The Origins of Soviet Biological Warfare* (Oxford: Oxford University Press, 2018).

138   Christopher J. Davis, "Nuclear Blindness: An Overview of the Biologi-
      cal Weapons Programs of the Former Soviet Union and Iraq," *Emerging
      Infectious Diseases* 5, no. 4 (1999): 509.
139   Robert Peterson, "Fear and Loathing in Moscow: The Russian Biological
      Weapons Program in 2022," *Bulletin of Atomic Scientists*, October 5, 2022,
      thebulletin.org/2022/10/the-russian-biological-weapons-program-in-2022.
140   Anthony Rimmington, *The Soviet Union's Invisible Weapons of Mass De-
      struction: Biopreparat's Covert Biological Warfare Programme* (Berlin:
      Springer Nature, 2021).
141   Jeanne Guillemin, "Scientists and the History of Biological Weapons: A
      Brief Historical Overview of the Development of Biological Weapons in
      the Twentieth Century," *EMBO Reports* 7, no. S1 (2006): S45–S49.
142   Rimmington, *Invisible Weapons*.
143   Ibid.
144   Ibid.
145   Ibid.
146   Zilinskas, *Soviet Biological Weapons*.
147   Ioannis Nikolakakis et al., "The History of Anthrax Weaponization in the
      Soviet Union," *Cureus* 15, no. 3 (2023).
148   Eliot Marshall, "Sverdlovsk: Anthrax Capital? Soviet Doctors Answer
      Questions About an Unusual Anthrax Epidemic Once Thought to Have
      Been Triggered by a Leak from a Weapons Lab," *Science* 240, no. 4851
      (1988): 383–85.
149   Matthew Meselson, "The Sverdlovsk Anthrax Outbreak of 1979," *Science*
      266, no. 5188 (1994): 1202–8.
150   Jeanne Guillemin, *Anthrax: The Investigation of a Deadly Outbreak* (Berkeley:
      University of California Press, 1999).
151   Ibid.
152   Ibid.
153   Jeanne Guillemin, "The 1979 Anthrax Epidemic in the USSR: Applied
      Science and Political Controversy," *Proceedings of the American Philosoph-
      ical Society* 146, no. 1 (2002): 18–36.
154   Ibid.

9. INFECTION AND THE BORDER, REVISITED

1   For a concise description of the Rio Grande, see "Rio Grande, in High De-
    mand," American Rivers, www.americanrivers.org/river/rio-grande; Rich-
    ard Griswold Del Castillo, *The Treaty of Guadalupe Hidalgo: A Legacy of
    Conflict* (Norman: University of Oklahoma Press, 1992).
2   Alice L. Baumgartner, *South to Freedom: Runaway Slaves to Mexico and the
    Road to the Civil War* (New York: Basic Books, 2020).

3   Baumgartner, *South to Freedom*. Also see a discussion of the book, John Burnett, "A Chapter in U.S. History Often Ignored: The Flight of Runaway Slaves to Mexico," *All Things Considered*, NPR, February 28, 2021, www.npr.org/2021/02/28/971325620/a-chapter-in-u-s-history-often -ignored-the-flight-of-runaway-slaves-to-mexico.

4   Baumgartner, *South to Freedom*.

5   Narrative of Former Slave Felix Haywood, 1936, https://www.npr.org /2021/02/28/971325620/a-chapter-in-u-s-history-often-ignored-the -flight-of-runaway-slaves-to-mexico

6   "Runaways: Selections from the WPA Interviews of Formerly Enslaved African Americans, 1936–1938," National Humanities Center Resource Toolbox, *The Making of African American Identity*, vol. 1, *1500–1965*, nationalhumanitiescenter.org/pds/maai/enslavement/text8/runawayswpa .pdf.

7   Russell Contreras, "Story of the Underground Railroad to Mexico Gains Attention," AP News, September 16, 2020, apnews.com/general-news-d2 6243702f11e27b59b591332bb6775e.

8   Baumgartner, *South to Freedom*.

9   For a description of the migration trail, its history, current challenges, and accounts of individuals, see Jason De León, *The Land of Open Graves: Living and Dying on the Migrant Trail*, vol. 36 (Berkeley: University of California Press, 2015).

10 Ibid.

11 ACLU, "Immigrants' Rights Advocates Release New Report Detailing Border Patrol's Inhumane Confiscations of Migrants' Personal Belongings," press release, February 12, 2024, www.aclu.org/press-releases/immigrants -rights-advocates-release-new-report-detailing-border-patrols-inhumane -confiscations-of-migrants-personal-belongings.

12 For a timeline of family separations up to 2022, see "Family Separation: A Timeline," Southern Poverty Law Center, March 23, 2022, www.splcenter .org/news/2022/03/23/family-separation-timeline. Family separations have continued under the Biden administration. See Mica Rosenberg, "The Biden Administration Is Separating Families at the Border. It Doesn't Always Say Why," *ProPublica*, December 12, 2024, www.propublica.org /article/family-separations-biden-russian-immigrants.

13 Video of the debate is available at www.youtube.com/watch?v=YsmgPp _nlok.

14 Transcript of the debate is available on the Reagan Library website: www.reaganlibrary.gov/archives/speech/1980-presidential-forum.

15 Jason De León, "1. Prevention Through Deterrence," in *The Land of Open Graves* (Berkeley: University of California Press, 2015), 21–37.

16 "The Cost of Immigration Enforcement and Border Security," American Immigration Council, August 2024, www.americanimmigrationcouncil .org/sites/default/files/research/cost_of_immigration_enforcement

_factsheet_2024.pdf; Douglas S. Massey, "The Counterproductive Consequences of Border Enforcement," *Cato Journal*, Fall 2017, www.cato.org /cato-journal/fall-2017/counterproductive-consequences-border -enforcement.

17 Roy Lubove, "The New Deal and National Health," *Current History* 45, no. 264 (1963): 77–117.

18 Lynne Page Snyder, "Passage and Significance of the 1944 Public Health Service Act," *Public Health Reports* 109, no. 6 (1994): 721.

19 Ibid.

20 Ibid.

21 Ibid.

22 Full text of Title 42 is available at www.law.cornell.edu/uscode/text/42.

23 42 U.S. Code § 265 Suspension of Entries and Imports from Designated Places to Prevent Spread of Communicable Diseases," www.law.cornell .edu/uscode/text/42/265.

24 For amendments to Title 42, see www.law.cornell.edu/uscode/text/42 /264.

25 Uriel Garcia, *Texas Tribune*, April 29, 2022, https://www.texastribune .org/2022/04/29/immigration-title-42-biden/.

26 Jason Dearen and Garance Burke, "Pence Ordered Borders Closed After CDC Experts Refused," AP News, October 3, 2020, apnews.com/article /virus-outbreak-pandemics-public-health-new-york-health-4ef0c6c5263 815a26f8aa17f6ea490ae.

27 Ibid.

28 Ibid.

29 Ibid.

30 Caitlin Dickerson and Michael Shear, "Before Covid-19, Trump Aide Sought to Use Disease to Close Borders," *New York Times*, May 3, 2020; Suzanne Monyak, "Top CDC Official Says Title 42 Border Policy 'Came from Outside,'" *Roll Call*, October 17, 2022, rollcall.com/2022/10/17 /top-cdc-official-says-title-42-border-policy-came-from-outside.

31 Ibid.

32 "Nationwide Enforcement Encounters: Title 8 Enforcement Actions and Title 42 Expulsions Fiscal Year 2022," U.S. Customs and Border Protection, www.cbp.gov/newsroom/stats/cbp-enforcement-statistics/title-8 -and-title-42-statistics-fy22.

33 Colleen Long, "Title 42 Has Ended. Here's What It Did, and How US Immigration Policy Is Changing," *AP News*, May 12, 2023, apnews.com /article/immigration-biden-border-title-42-mexico-asylum-be4e0b15b27 adb9bede87b9bbefb798d.

34 Morgan Sandhu, "Unprecedented Expulsion of Immigrants at the Southern Border: The Title 42 Process," The Petrie-Flow Center, December 26, 2020, blog.petrieflom.law.harvard.edu/2020/12/26/title-42-expulsion-of -immigrants.

35   Camilo Montoya-Galvez, "What Is Title 42, the COVID Border Policy Used to Expel Migrants?," *CBS News*, January 2, 2023, www.cbsnews.com /news/title-42-immigration-border-biden-covid-19-cdc.

36   Kathryn Hampton, Michele Heisler, Cynthia Pompa, and Alana Slavin, "Neither Safety nor Health: How Title 42 Expulsions Harm Health and Violate Rights," Physicians for Human Rights, July 28, 2021, phr.org/our -work/resources/neither-safety-nor-health.

37   Kathryn Hampton, Michele Heisler, Cynthia Pompa, and Alana Slavin, "Neither Safety nor Health: How Title 42 Expulsions Harm Health and Violate Rights," Physicians for Human Rights, July 28, 2021, phr.org/our -work/resources/neither-safety-nor-health.

38   Ibid.

39   Ibid.

40   Denise N. Obinna, "Title 42 and the Power to Exclude: Asylum Seekers and the Denial of Entry into the United States," *Politics and Policy* 51, no. 4 (2023): 508–23.

41   Joseph Nwadiuko and Arturo Vargas Bustamante, "Little to No Corre-lation Found Between Immigrant Entry and COVID-19 Infection Rates in the United States: Study Examines the Correlation Between Immigrant Entry into the US and COVID-19 Infections Rates," *Health Affairs* 41, no. 11 (2022): 1635–44.

42   Hampton, "Neither Safety nor Health."

43   Hampton, "Neither Safety nor Health"; Michael R. Ulrich and Sondra S. Crosby, "42, Asylum, and Politicising Public Health," *Lancet Regional Health–Americas* 7 (2022).

44   "White House Criticizes Border Agents Who Rounded Up Migrants on Horseback," *The Guardian*, September 20, 2021, www.theguardian.com /us-news/2021/sep/20/us-begins-deportation-flights-haitians-texas -border-town.

45   John Burnett, "Judge Says Coronavirus Can't Be Used as Reason to Quickly Deport Unaccompanied Minors," NPR, November 18, 2020, www.npr .org/2020/11/18/936312918/judge-says-coronavirus-cant-be-used-as -reason-to-deport-unaccompanied-minors.

46   John Gramlich, "Key Facts About Title 42, the Pandemic Policy That Has Reshaped Immigration Enforcement at U.S.-Mexico Border," Pew Re-search Center, April 27, 2022, www.pewresearch.org/short-reads/2022 /04/27/key-facts-about-title-42-the-pandemic-policy-that-has-reshaped -immigration-enforcement-at-u-s-mexico-border.

47   Jasmine Aguilera, "Biden Is Expelling Migrants on COVID-19 Grounds But Health Experts Say That's All Wrong," *Time*, October 12, 2021, time .com/6105055/biden-title-42-covid-19.

48   Ibid.

49   Camilo Montoya-Galvez, "Top CDC Scientist Said COVID-Era Health Policy Used to Expel Migrants Unfairly Stigmatized Them," *CBS News*,

November 21, 2022, www.cbsnews.com/news/top-cdc-scientist-said-covid
-era-health-policy-used-to-expel-migrants-unfairly-stigmatized-them.

50   Jasmine Aguilera, "Biden Is Expelling Migrants on COVID-19 Grounds
but Health Experts Say That's All Wrong," *Time*, October 12, 2021, time
.com/6105055/biden-title-42-covid-19.

51   Julia Ainsley, "Biden Administration to Lift Title 42 Covid Restriction on
Border in May Officials Say," *NBC News*, March 20, 2022, www.nbcnews
.com/politics/immigration/biden-admin-lift-title-42-covid-restriction
-border-may-officials-say-rcna22278.

52   Rebecca Beitsch and Rafael Bernal, "Vulnerable Senate Democrats Un-
dercut Biden on Title 42," *The Hill*, April 7, 2022, thehill.com/latino
/3261056-vulnerable-senate-democrats-undercut-biden-on-title-42.

53   Megan Barth, "Sen. Cortez Masto Flip Flops on Title 42," *Nevada Globe*,
April 7, 2022, thenevadaglobe.com/congress/sen-cortez-masto-flip-flops
-on-title-42.

54   Rebecca Beitsch and Rafael Bernal, "Vulnerable Senate Democrats Un-
dercut Biden on Title 42," *The Hill*, April 7, 2022, thehill.com/latino
/3261056-vulnerable-senate-democrats-undercut-biden-on-title-42.

55   Raja Razek and Devan Cole, "GOP-Led States Sue Over Decision to
End Trump-Era Pandemic Restrictions at the US Border," CNN, April 4,
2022, edition.cnn.com/2022/04/04/politics/republican-states-lawsuit
-biden-administration-title-42/index.html.

56   Muzaffar Chishti, Kathleen Bush-Joseph, and Julian Montalvo, "Title 42
Postmortem: U.S. Pandemic-Era Expulsions Policy Did Not Shut Down
the Border," Migration Policy Institute, April 25, 2024, www.migration
policy.org/article/title-42-autopsy; Ashley Niles, "Migrant Health After
the End of Title 42," *Think Global Health*, July 26, 2023, www.thinkglobal
health.org/article/migrant-health-after-end-title-42.

57   Dominick Mastrangelo, "Fauci: Immigrants 'Absolutely Not' Driving
Coronavirus Infections in US," *The Hill*, October 4, 2021, thehill.com
/policy/healthcare/public-global-health/575123-fauci-immigrants
-absolutely-not-driving-coronavirus.

58   Anne G. Beckett, Loune Viaud, Michele Heisler, and Joia Mukherjee,
"Misusing Public Health as a Pretext to End Asylum—Title 42," *New
England Journal of Medicine* 386, no. 16 (2022): e41; Rachel Fabi, Saul D.
Rivas, and Marsha Griffin, "Not in Our Name: The Disingenuous Use of
'Public Health' as Justification for Title 42 Expulsions in the Era of the
Migrant Protection Protocols," *American Journal of Public Health* 112,
no. 8 (2022): 1115–19.

59   "CBP Issues Memo on Title 42 Exceptions for Ukrainian Nationals,"
American Immigration Lawyers Association, March 11, 2022 (US Customs and Border Protection. Title 42 Exceptions for Ukrainian Nationals),
www.aila.org/library/cbp-issues-memo-on-title-42-exceptions.

60   Jill Garamone, "Military Phase of Evacuation Ends as Does America's
     Longest War," *DOD News*, August 30, 2021, www.defense.gov/news/news
     -stories/article/article/2759031/military-phase-of-evacuation-ends-as
     -does-americas-longest-war.
61   D. Parvaz, "Since the Taliban Takeover Afghans Hoping to Leave
     Afghanistan Have Few Ways Out," NPR, October 3, 2022, www.npr.org
     /2022/10/03/1121053865/afghanistan-refugees-visas.
62   Umar Farooq, "Afghan Neighbours Wary of New Refugee Crisis as
     Violence Surges," Reuters, July 15, 2021, www.reuters.com/world/asia
     -pacific/afghan-neighbours-wary-new-refugee-crisis-violence-surges
     -2021-07-15.
63   Muhammad H. Zaman, *We Wait for a Miracle: Healthcare and the Forcibly
     Displaced* (Baltimore: Johns Hopkins University Press, 2023).
64   Ibid.
65   Alisha Saleem, Maha Rashid, Ameerah Shaikh, and Sajjad Ali, "Lack of
     COVID-19 Vaccination in Rural Areas of Pakistan," *Vacunas* 23 (2022):
     S125–S126.
66   Anwar Iqbal, "US Wants Pakistan to Keep Afghan Border Open for
     DPs," *Dawn News*, August 5, 2021, www.dawn.com/news/1638887.

10. WEAPONIZING THE SHIELD

1   "War and Infectious Diseases: Brothers in Arms," *Lancet Infectious Dis-
    eases* 22, no. 5 (2022): 563.
2   M.M. Manring, Alan Hawk, Jason H. Calhoun, and Romney C. Andersen,
    "Treatment of War Wounds: A Historical Review," *Clinical Orthopaedics
    and Related Research* 467 (2009): 2168–91.
3   Clinton K. Murray, Mary K. Hinkle, and Heather C. Yun, "History of
    Infections Associated with Combat-Related Injuries," *Journal of
    Trauma and Acute Care Surgery* 64, no. 3 (2008): S221–31.
4   Manring et al., "Treatment of War Wounds."
5   Richard D. Forrest, "Development of Wound Therapy from the Dark Ages
    to the Present," *Journal of the Royal Society of Medicine* 75, no. 4 (1982):
    268–73.
6   Paul Weindling, "Health and Medicine in Interwar Europe," in *Medicine
    in the Twentieth Century*, ed. Roger Cooter and John V. Pickstone (London:
    Taylor and Francis, 2020), 39–50.
7   Thomas Schlich and Bruno J. Strasser, "Making the Medical Mask: Sur-
    gery, Bacteriology, and the Control of Infection (1870s–1920s)," *Medical
    History* 66, no. 2 (2022): 116–34.
8   For discussion of Fleming's discovery, the history, the legend, and the
    myths, see Robert Bud, *Penicillin: Triumph and Tragedy* (Oxford: Oxford

University Press, 2007); Eric Lax, *The Mould in Dr Florey's Coat* (Little, Brown, 2004); Kevin Brown, *Penicillin Man* (Gloucestershire: History Press, 2005); William Rosen, *Miracle Cure: The Creation of Antibiotics and the Birth of Modern Medicine* (New York: Penguin, 2017); Muhammad H. Zaman, *Biography of Resistance* (New York: HarperCollins, 2020).

9   John E. Lesch, ed. *The First Miracle Drugs: How the Sulfa Drugs Transformed Medicine* (Oxford: Oxford University Press, 2006).

10   Ibid.

11   "Medicine: Prontosil," *Time*, December 28, 1936, time.com/archive /6769481/medicine-prontosil.

12   Zaman, *Biography of Resistance.*

13   Ibid.

14   For the development of penicillin at the Dunn School, see Ronald Bentley, "The Development of Penicillin: Genesis of a Famous Antibiotic," *Perspectives in Biology and Medicine* 48, no. 3 (2005): 444–52; Bud, *Penicillin*; Lax, *Mould in Dr Florey's Coat*; Brown, *Penicillin Man*; Rosen, *Miracle Cure*; Zaman, *Biography of Resistance.*

15   Albert Alexander's story was recently shared again by members of his family. See Michael Barrett, "The Legacy of Penicillin's First Patient; Albert Alexander's Story Should Inspire Us to Renew Humanity's Struggle Against Antimicrobial Resistant Infections," *New Statesman*, June 27, 2023, www.newstatesman.com/politics/health/2023/06/albert-alexander -legacy-penicillin-first-patient.

16   Peter Neushul, "Science, Government and the Mass Production of Penicillin," *Journal of the History of Medicine and Allied Sciences* 48, no. 4 (1993): 371–95.

17   Ibid.

18   For the NRRL work, see Bud, *Penicillin: Triumph and Tragedy.*

19   William Rosen, *Miracle Cure*; Zaman, *Biography of Resistance.*

20   Ibid.

21   Ibid.

22   Robert Gaynes, "The Discovery of Penicillin—New Insights After More than 75 Years of Clinical Use," *Emerging Infectious Diseases* 23, no. 5 (2017): 849.

23   Peter Neushul, "Science, Government and the Mass Production of Penicillin," *Journal of the History of Medicine and Allied Sciences* 48, no. 4 (1993): 371–95.

24   Rosen, *Miracle Cure.*

25   Ibid.

26   Neushul, "Mass Production of Penicillin."

27   Gaynes, "Discovery of Penicillin."

28   Ibid.

29   Ibid.

30   "'Thanks to Penicillin ... He Will Come Home!' The Challenge of Mass Production," National WWII Museum, www.nationalww2museum.org /sites/default/files/2017-07/thanks-to-penicillin-lesson.pdf.

31   Ibid.

32   Some examples available at exhibits.lib.usu.edu/items/show/18775; Andrew Adiletta, *Penicillin: How World War II Affected the Public Reception of the World's Most Influential Drug* (paper, Worcester Polytechnic Institute, 2022), https://www.researchgate.net/publication/369997851 _Penicillin_How_World_War_II_Affected_the_Public_Reception_of _The_World%27s_Most_Influential_Drug.

33   Alexa Heathorn and Sara Slagle, "Penicillin and Pneumonia," in *Science, Technology, and Society: A Student-Led Exploration* (Clemson, SC: Clemson University, 2020), pressbooks.pub/anne1/chapter/penicillin -and-pneumonia.

34   Robert Bud, "Penicillin and the New Elizabethans," *British Journal for the History of Science* 31, no. 3 (1998): 305–33.

35   Zaman, *Biography of Resistance.*

36   Ibid.

37   Ibid.

38   Marc Landas, *Cold War Resistance: The International Struggle over Antibiotics* (Lincoln: University of Nebraska Press, 2020).

39   Michael L. Hoffman, "U.N. Health Body Seeks U.S. Penicillin Aid for Soviet Bloc, Which Charges Embargo," *New York Times*, March 3, 1949, www.nytimes.com/1949/03/03/archives/un-health-body-seeks-us -penicillin-aid-for-soviet-bloc-which.html.

40   Ibid.

41   Ibid.

42   Mauro Capocci, "Cold Drugs: Circulation, Production and Intelligence of Antibiotics in Post-WWII Years," *Medicina nei Secoli: Journal of History of Medicine and Medical Humanities* 26, no. 2 (2014): 401–22.

43   Ibid.

44   No. 147: *Memorandum of Discussion at the 169th Meeting of the National Security Council, Washington, November 5, 1953,* Eisenhower Library, Eisenhower papers, Whitman file, Office of the Historian, history.state .gov/historicaldocuments/frus1952-54v14p1/d147.

45   Ibid.

46   Capocci, "Cold Drugs."

47   Jeanne Guillemin, *Biological Weapons: From the Invention of State-Sponsored Programs to Contemporary Bioterrorism* (New York: Columbia University Press, 2005).

48   Nicole Boardman, "Global Allocation of the COVID-19 Vaccine and Its Ethical Implications," Markkula Center for Applied Ethics, February 11, 2021, www.scu.edu/ethics/healthcare-ethics-blog/global-allocation-of -the-covid-19-vaccine-and-its-ethical-implications.

49   Nurith Aizenman, "Low Income Nations Need COVID Vaccines. Rich Countries Have Millions of Unused Doses," *All Things Considered*, NPR, November 8, 2021, www.npr.org/2021/11/08/1053647185/low-income -nations-need-covid-vaccines-rich-countries-have-millions-of-unused-do.

50   Francesco Guarascio, "Poorer Nations Reject over 100 Mln COVID-19 Vaccine Doses as Many Near Expiry," Reuters, January 14, 2022, www .reuters.com/business/healthcare-pharmaceuticals/more-than-100-million -covid-19-vaccines-rejected-by-poorer-nations-dec-unicef-2022-01-13.

51   Brenice Duroseau, Nodar Kipshidze, and Rupali Jayant Limaye, "The Impact of Delayed Access to COVID-19 Vaccines in Low- and Lower-Middle-Income Countries," *Frontiers in Public Health* 10 (2023): 1087138.

52   Antonia Farzan and Helosia Traiano, "U.S. Officials Pushed Brazil to Reject Russia's Coronavirus Vaccine, According to HHS Report," *Washington Post*, March 16, 2021; Chris Bing and Joel Schectman, "Pentagon Ran Secret Anti-vax Campaign to Undermine China During Pandemic," Reuters, June 14, 2024, www.reuters.com/investigates/special -report/usa-covid-propaganda.

CONCLUSION

1   James W. Curran and Harold W. Jaffe, "AIDS: The Early Years and CDC's Response," Morbidity and Mortality Weekly Report (MMWR) *Surveillance Summaries* 60, no. suppl 4 (2011): 64–69.

2   Ibid.

3   For a timeline of HIV, see HIV.gov, www.hiv.gov/hiv-basics/overview /history/hiv-and-aids-timeline#year-1981.

4   Lawrence Altman, "New Homosexual Disorder Worries Health Officials," *New York Times*, May 11, 1982.

5   See HIV.gov, www.hiv.gov/hiv-basics/overview/history/hiv-and-aids -timeline#year-1982.

6   German Lopez, "The Reagan Administration's Unbelievable Response to the HIV/AIDS Epidemic," *Vox*, December 1, 2016, www.vox.com /2015/12/1/9828348/ronald-reagan-hiv-aids.

7   See HIV timeline, www.hiv.gov/hiv-basics/overview/history/hiv-and -aids-timeline#year-1982.

8   Federal Response to AIDS: Hearings Before a Subcommittee of the Committee on Government Operations House of Representatives Ninety-Eighth Congress First Session August 1 and 2 1983. https://li.proquest .com/elhpdf/histcontext/HRG-1983-OPH-0054.pdf.

9   HIV timeline, www.hiv.gov/hiv-basics/overview/history/hiv-and-aids -timeline#year-1982.

10   Lopez, "Unbelievable Response."

11   Dudley Clendinen, "Aids Spreads Pain and Fear Among Ill and Healthy Alike," *New York Times*, June 17, 1983.

12   Alison Patterson, *Institutional Negligence: The AIDS Crisis in 1980s America* (Providence College, December 15, 2017), digitalcommons.providence.edu/cgi/viewcontent.cgi?article=1002&context=history_undergrad_theses.

13   Frank Pellegrini, "Fool on the Hill," *Time*, May 8, 1998.

14   Patterson, *Institutional Negligence*.

15   David W. Purcell, "Forty Years of HIV: The Intersection of Laws, Stigma, and Sexual Behavior and Identity," *American Journal of Public Health* 111, no. 7 (2021): 1231–33.

16   Transcript of the speech of September 16, 1985, www.reaganlibrary.gov/archives/speech/presidents-news-conference-16.

17   Philip M. Boffey, "Reagan Urges Wide Aids Testing but Does Not Call for Compulsion," *New York Times*, June 1, 1987.

18   HIV timeline, www.hiv.gov/hiv-basics/overview/history/hiv-and-aids-timeline#year-1982.

19   HIV statistics, www.hiv.gov/hiv-basics/overview/data-and-trends/statistics.

20   US Federal Funding for HIV/AIDS: Trends Over Time," KFF, March 26, 2024, www.kff.org/hivaids/fact-sheet/u-s-federal-funding-for-hivaids-trends-over-time.

21   Richard Parker, "Grassroots Activism, Civil Society Mobilization, and the Politics of the Global HIV/AIDS Epidemic," *Brown Journal of World Affairs* 17 (2010): 21.

22   For detailed statistics, see "What Is the Impact of HIV on Racial and Ethnic Minorities in the U.S.?," HIV.gov, October 8, 2024, www.hiv.gov/hiv-basics/overview/data-and-trends/impact-on-racial-and-ethnic-minorities.

23   For a discussion of new technologies and their impact on vulnerable communities, see Petra Molnar, *The Walls Have Eyes: Surviving Migration in the Age of Artificial Intelligence* (New York: The New Press, 2024).

24   Xiaolong Hou, Yang Jiao, Leilei Shen, and Zhuo Chen, "The Lasting Impact of the Tuskegee Syphilis Study: COVID-19 Vaccination Hesitation Among African Americans," *Journal of Population Economics* 37, no. 2 (2024): 41.

Index

About the Author

Muhammad H. Zaman is an award-winning educator and researcher at Boston University, where he is Howard Hughes Medical Institute Professor of Biomedical Engineering and International Health. He is the author of *Biography of Resistance: The Epic Battle Between People and Pathogens.* He lives in Boston.

Publishing in the Public Interest

Thank you for reading this book published by The New Press; we hope you enjoyed it. New Press books and authors play a crucial role in sparking conversations about the key political and social issues of our day.

We hope that you will stay in touch with us. To keep up to date with our books, events, and the issues we cover, follow us on social media and sign up for our newsletter at thenewpress.org.

Please consider buying New Press books not only for yourself, but also for friends and family and to donate to schools, libraries, community centers, prison libraries, and other organizations involved with the issues our authors write about.

The New Press is a 501(c)(3) nonprofit organization; if you wish to support our work with a tax-deductible gift please visit https://thenewpress.org/donate/ or use the QR code below.